Neurologic-Psychiatric Syndromes in Focus

Part I – From Neurology to Psychiatry

Frontiers of Neurology and Neuroscience

Vol. 41

Neurologic-Psychiatric Syndromes in Focus

Part I – From Neurology to Psychiatry

Vol. 42

Neurologic-Psychiatric Syndromes in Focus

Part II – From Psychiatry to Neurology

Series Editor

J. Bogousslavsky Montreux

Neurologic-Psychiatric Syndromes in Focus

Part I – From Neurology to Psychiatry

Volume Editor

J. Bogousslavsky Montreux

16 figures, 5 in color, and 6 tables, 2018

KARGER Basel · Freiburg · Paris · London · New York · Chennai · New Delhi · Bangkok · Beijing · Shanghai · Tokyo · Kuala Lumpur · Singapore · Sydney

Frontiers of Neurology and Neuroscience
Vols. 1–18 were published as Monographs in Clinical Neuroscience

---

Julien Bogousslavsky, MD
Head, Neurocenter, Swiss Medical Network
Geneva-Genolier-Lausanne-Montreux-
Neuchatel-Fribourg-Lugano-Basel-Zurich
Clinique Valmont, CH–1823 Glion (Switzerland)

Library of Congress Cataloging-in-Publication Data

Names: Bogousslavsky, Julien, editor.
Title: Neurologic-psychiatric syndromes in focus / volume editor, J. Bogousslavsky.
Other titles: Frontiers of neurology and neuroscience ; v. 41-42. 1660-4431
Description: Basel ; New York : Karger, [2018] | Series: Frontiers of neurology and neuroscience, ISSN 1660-4431 ; vol. 41-42 | Includes bibliographical references and index.
Identifiers: LCCN 2017044042| ISBN 9783318058581 (v. 1 : alk. paper) | ISBN 9783318060881 (v. 2 : alk. paper) | ISBN 9783318058598 (v. 1 electronic version) | ISBN 9783318060898 (v. 2 electronic version)
Subjects: | MESH: Brain Diseases--complications | Mental Disorders--etiology | Neurobehavioral Manifestations
Classification: LCC RC454.4 | NLM WL 348 | DDC 616.89/071--dc23 LC record available at https://lccn.loc.gov/2017044042

Bibliographic Indices. This publication is listed in bibliographic services, including Current Contents® and Index Medicus.

www.karger.com
Printed on acid-free and non-aging paper (ISO 9706)
ISSN 1660–4431
e-ISSN 1662–2804
ISBN 978–3–318–05858–1
e-ISBN 978–3–318–05859–8

Contents

Introduction

The late 19th century and early 20th century witnessed neurology and psychiatry becoming two distinct fields in medicine. However, many overlaps between the two fields have been since then, leading to the reactivation of the clinical approach, thought to mainly bear a historical relevance. Neurologists have now become interested in mood and behavior, because they observed that emotional behavioral changes were often dramatically significant in patients with focal brain lesions or neurodegenerative disorders. On the contrary, psychiatrists have developed a renewed interest in the brain and its interaction with the psychological state. It is striking that while "neuropsychiatry" progressively became obsolete during the second half of the 20th century, a new approach to the functional changes associated with brain lesions and to the cerebral correlates of psychological dysfunction may justify a modern redefinition of the field.

Many neurologic-psychiatric syndromes have remained poorly known, because of a rarity in the literature which could often be explained by their position in the former no-man's-land between classical neurology and psychiatry. The goal of the present book, which is divided into two parts (for Part II – From Psychiatry to Neurology, see Frontiers of Neurology and Neuroscience, vol. 42), is to shed light on the so-called "uncommon syndromes," which may in fact be more frequent than what the literature suggests. Since several of these clinical syndromes were first reported over a century ago, they are often known by an eponym (Ganser, Capgras, de Cérambault, Cotard, etc.) or a mythological or fictional figure (Diogenes, Othello, Alice in Wonderland, etc.). This also explains why the historical description and development of these neuropsychiatric syndromes is of particular interest, and we have attempted to give details on this perspective across time. We have also tried to focus on the most representative clinical syndromes, excluding from our survey very common manifestations (anosognosia, confabulation) which have been the specific topic of recent reviews, or particular forms of delusions (delusional parasitosis) which do not bring specific information as compared to other delusional syndromes covered here.

Dr. Julien Bogousslavsky

Bogousslavsky J (ed): Neurologic-Psychiatric Syndromes in Focus. Part I – From Neurology to Psychiatry.
Front Neurol Neurosci. Basel, Karger, 2018, vol 41, pp 1–13 (DOI: 10.1159/000475690)

Minor Hemisphere Major Syndromes

Antonio Carota[a] · Julien Bogousslavsky[b]

[a]Clinique de Genolier, Genolier, and [b]Neurocenter, Swiss Medical Network, Clinique Valmont, Glion/Montreux, Switzerland

Abstract

A right "minor hemisphere" does not exist as the right hemisphere is dominant for awareness (nosognosia), spatial attention, emotional regulation, facial and voice expressions, visual recognition, and topographical orientation. Without the right hemisphere, the world would be flat, deprived of general and spatial attentions, pointing preferentially to the right side of the space, lacking visual experiences and emotions, exhibiting diminished awareness of the self and environment. Clinical-related syndromes of the right hemisphere are unilateral spatial neglect, object and face visual agnosia, the anosognosia for hemiparesis and/or hemianopia, misidentification syndromes, mania, and other obsessions for the food and the body. Another key function of the right hemisphere is the modulation of the emotional processes of the linguistic communication (as prosody and facial expressions), and the tuning of some holistic aspects of language as the understanding of the abstract and figurative characters. The great mysteries of the right brain hemisphere concern the origin of the emotional nature of the human being, the way by which cognition interacts with perception and finally the human consciousness. Multidisciplinary researches in the domains of neurology, cognitive psychology, neuropsychiatry, functional neuroimaging, and neurophysiology will reveal in the future some of these mysteries.

Introduction

The left hemisphere has been the first object of clinical and cognitive researches since the first half of the 19th century, as early as it began evident that the aphasic syndromes were associated to left hemisphere lesions in specific language areas. Hence, the left brain became the hemisphere dominant for language.

Unfortunately, these early studies contributed to create a rivalry of the 2 hemispheres. The existence of conflicting or regulatory actions (the tonic inhibition theory) that one hemisphere carries out at detriment of the other throughout the corpus

Table 1. Specific syndromes which are the signature of the dysfunction of the right hemisphere

Unilateral spatial neglect
Constructional apraxia
Dressing apraxia
Hypergraphia
Visuoperceptive syndromes
Object agnosia
Prosopagnosia
Topographical disorientation
Communicative deficits
Dysprosody
Neuropsychiatric syndromes
Anosognosia and somatognosia
Misidentification syndromes
Mania

callosum (the main brain inter-hemispheric commissure containing 200 millions of fibers) was, in the 1960s and 1970s, the object of dichotic and tachistoscopic studies in "split-brain" (commissurotomized) patients [1].

These studies showed the dominant role of the right hemisphere for attention and visual perception, and this dominance found confirmation from clinical studies on the right hemisphere syndromes surging after stroke (i.e., spatial neglect, anosognosia for hemiparesis, and visual agnosias [VA]).

In the end of the 20th century, neuropsychological studies focused on the cognitive mechanisms of those syndromes.

Since the beginning of the last century, because of the diffusion of functional neuroimaging, the scientific interest shifted to the integrative functions of the hemispheres. Now, the aim is to define resting states [2], activation patterns, connectivity, neural networks, and diaschisis phenomena. The interest is on the mechanisms of recovery or compensation adopted by the homolog areas of the opposite hemisphere too.

In this chapter, we mainly discuss the stroke syndromes of the right hemisphere (Table 1) as their clinical manifestation are usually more flamboyant, and their incidence is higher than with other diseases. However, the same syndromes could associate with developmental, neurodegenerative, and inflammatory diseases of the brain, brain cancer, and trauma.

Disease Pathogenesis

Unilateral Spatial Neglect

Unilateral spatial neglect (USN) is defined as a cluster of symptoms and signs, suggesting a failure to orient or react to stimuli located on the side of the space opposite to the lesion (usually on the left side in case of the right hemisphere damage) [3]. Primary sensory or motor deficits should be excluded as the cause of USN-like behaviors. Generally, USN patients do not have or have only partial awareness of the syndrome. Post-stroke USN incidence varies from 20 to 80% following right hemisphere stroke and 5–10% after left hemisphere stroke. This large variance in incidence depends principally from the instruments employed for assessment (pencil-paper tests generally). Computerized tests measuring response times (in milliseconds) are undoubtedly the most accurate for USN detection as they allow the most precise statistical analyses, and would also detect minor signs [4]. Behavioral signs are also diagnostic as the left asymmetry for hanging spectacles or grooming. There is evidence that patients with USN can also distort toward the right side of the number line [5] and temporal events too [6] as if they were located in a spatial array ("what is before is the left").

USN is a heterogeneous syndrome (Table 2), which also includes rare and not yet sufficiently explained sensory phenomena such as allesthesia (misperception of the location side of a stimulus), allochiria (response to stimuli presented to one side of their body as if the stimuli had been presented at the opposite side), asomatognosia (loss of recognition or awareness of a limb), and other illusory sensory misperceptions (as the feeling that the plegic limb is larger or longer), USN-related blind sight (responses to visual stimuli that are neglected on the left side), anosognosia of USN (incapacity of the patient to be partially or fully aware of the condition of USN) [7].

Furthermore, USN associates with even rarer and productive "psychiatric-visuoperceptive" phenomena (perseverations, confabulations, false beliefs, misidentifications), illusory limb movements (the belief to have moved the paralyzed limb), supernumerary limbs (the illusion of multiple limbs on the weak side), somatoparaphrenia (the denial of the ownership of a limb which is attributed to another person), and misoplegia (morbidly hating or disliking the plegic limb, identified as the "devil" [personal observation]).

This heterogeneity of the USN phenomena depends on the lesion extension and location, the time elapsed since stroke, and different compensation mechanisms acting during the recovery phase. The general level of arousal and non-spatial attention deficits could also explain the large fluctuations of the USN severity.

Thus, the USN assessment should take into account all the USN variants and related phenomena to construct a specific patient's profile. This is the only means to understand more profitably the role of the lesion and to plan correct rehabilitation programs.

The brain network supporting the functions of spatial attention includes the temporoparietal junction, the inferior parietal lobule, the angular and supramarginal gyrus, the premotor frontal 44, 6, and 8 areas, the medial and lateral temporal lobe, the cingular gyrus, the pulvinar, and superior colliculus [8]. Lesions of the basal ganglia and the internal capsule could also determine or influence USN.

Table 2. Types of USN

Visual USN
According to spatial coordinates
Egocentric
Retinal axis
Head axis
Trunk axis
Limb axis
Allocentric
Environment-based USN
Object-based USN
Gravity axis
Next space
–Personal space
–Peripersonal space
Far space
Mental space (representational USN)
Other sensory modalities
Auditory USN
Tactile USN
Olfactory USN
Gustatory USN
Motor USN
Hypokinesia
Hypometria
Directional hypokinesia
Motor impersistence
USN-related phenomena
Extinction to double stimulation
Allochiria
Blindsight and unconscious perception
Anosognosia

The theories on the mechanisms of USN should take into account all the USN variants, explain the role of the lesion of the right hemisphere, the attraction toward the ipsilesional side, the presence of USN signs also in the ipsilesional space, and the link between visual and "representational" neglect [9], this last condition being independent of external stimuli.

A unitary theory of USN seems invalid. A unique deficit of spatial attention for which the right hemisphere is undoubtedly dominant could not explain the other USN phenomena, such as emotional changes (blunted affect), changes in self-awareness (e.g. anosognosia of neurologic deficits including USN itself), and related "perceptive-psychiatric" phenomena. We should study the USN in tridimensional spaces and in daily life activities outside the hospitals, controlling at the same time, the respective role of mental and physical (next and far spaces, ego, and allocentric coordinates) frames of reference.

The internal and external distortions of motor, sensitive, and spatial frames occurring with USN force us to think the USN-related world as an inhuman or alien universe.

Many rehabilitative programs exist for USN (essentially distinct in the bottom-up or top-down categories). The effect of such interventions to improve USN in daily life activities and in the long-term is still the object of controversies.

Constructional Apraxia

Kleist (1934) first defined constructional apraxia (CA) as the deficit of reproducing the correct spatial configuration of objects by drawing or assembling their parts. However, such a deficit should not be the consequence of a primary sensory failure or USN. Indeed, a thoughtful analysis of the paintings of famous artists after right brain damage showed that USN and CA almost completely dissociate [10].

Drawing or assembling objects depends on several brain functions (sustained attention, reasoning, spatial planning, sensory and graphomotor abilities, visual working memory, and spatial coding). Drawing by memory can also use non-spatial or verbal resources. For this reason, it is difficult to categorize CA into specific subtypes. CA is probably and primarily a spatial deficit, as the patient does not reproduce the spatial relations of the elements of the objects because he or she does not understand them.

It is difficult to define the epidemiological incidence of this disorder for either vascular or degenerative diseases, as it is not routinely evaluated with specific test.

The assessment of CA includes drawing and assembling tests of unfamiliar objects (such as complex figures) to avoid cultural effects. However, the copy of such figures also requires the elaboration of high graphomotor strategies that depend on the frontal lobe. The patients with right hemisphere lesions have the tendency to distort the whole object, while the patients with left hemisphere lesions tend to simplify or omit the details with the result of an oversimplification [11]. Patients with dementia produce more graphic perseverations than patients with right hemisphere stroke, and exhibit the "closing-in" phenomenon, which is a sort of clinical signature (with rare exceptions) of the Alzheimer's disease [12].

CA manifests with frontal and parietal lesions, and more rarely with basal ganglia and thalamic lesions, with some clinical differences, such as a more pronounced visual spatial deficit with posterior lesions and a more motor programming dysfunction with anterior lesions [13]. There are no unified rehabilitation programs for CA.

Dressing Apraxia

Dressing apraxia (DA) indicates the inability to orient and adjust the clothes to the body, after excluding that this difficulty is due mainly to primary motor and sensory deficit or to a global cognitive deterioration (as dementia), or uniquely to USN. DA, as well as CA, as a consequence of right hemisphere damage, are preeminently a spatial disorder [14]. No definite epidemiological data exists for this disorder.

DA manifests with behaviors of perplexity, passivity and with stereotyped, uncoordinated or dispersed acts. The clinical evaluation consists of asking the subject to dress himself, or to dress a dummy or a doll. For research purposes, all the patients should be examined under the same conditions and preferably filmed. As well as CA, DA is related to right frontal and parietal lesions, and is often associated to USN [15].

Rehabilitation of dressing apraxia could be particularly difficult, especially if the patient has reduced insight of the condition.

Hypergraphia

Hypergraphia (HG), a compulsive writing behavior, due to stroke on the right hemisphere, is very different from that associated with temporal lobe epilepsy and characterized by detailed and meaningful writing. Indeed, the main features of post-stroke HG are spatial distortions, graphic perseverations, letter and down stroke omissions, discourse incoherence, rupture of grammatical and syntactical rules.

Post-stroke HG is an extremely rare syndrome, mostly described with frontal, parietal or cingular lesions [16, 17].

Visual Agnosia

VA defines the difficulty of recognizing the objects only by the visual modality, after excluding that this failure could be due to aphasia, USN or dementia. Although this syndrome is generally consequent to bilateral occipital-parietal stroke, a unilateral right lesion would be sufficient for VA to manifest. Thus, the right hemisphere plays a dominant role in computing the shapes and spatial coordinates of the objects.

VA is a rare condition, occurring with 1–5% of stroke of the posterior cerebral artery [18]. The prevalence would be probably much higher if standardized batteries of visual recognition were used for assessment.

Developmental cases and specific degenerative diseases such as posterior cortical atrophy, can manifest with a pure form of the condition.

VA could be distinct coarsely in the apperceptive (apVA) and associative (asVA) variants, a distinction proposed by Lissauer in 1890, more than a century ago.

The apVA is a visual recognition deficit intervening at the stage of the elaboration of the sensory elemental characteristics of the objects. It could be further distinguished in other subtypes: agnosia for shapes or "visual form" agnosia [19], agnosia for perspectives, and an integrative form of agnosia (inability to integrate the details in the global form, the condition of, metaphorically speaking, "seeing the trees but not the forest") [20].

Very rare cases of "mirror agnosia" or agnosia for mirror stimuli (the condition of confusing the mirror image of an object with a real object) have been reported and related to posterior parietal lesions on the right hemisphere [21–23].

The diagnosis of apVA requires checking that defects of luminosity perception, movement perception (akinetopsia), color discrimination (achromatopsia), and visual and semantic memories are not the main causes of visual dysfunction. Patients with VA generally show spared abilities of visual imagery. They remember the objects that they could not copy or recognize visually. The Birmingham object recognition battery is a useful tool of assessment as it allows analyzing accurately the perceptive and semantic abilities necessary for object recognition.

One of the first case reports of VA was that of a woman entirely unable to recognize visually the objects but able to grab them rapidly and with correct hand orientation.

This seminal case suggested the existence of 2 different neural networks within the right hemisphere – the dual stream hypothesis [24] – related to recognition (the ventral stream) and to object-related actions (the dorsal stream).

Several experimental studies on human and primates provided evidence of this functional dissociation in recognition processes.

Finally, the right hemisphere would be specialized for integrating the elemental characteristics of the object (shapes, orientation, and contours) and its perspective to compare them with an object prototype, which is stocked in the memory system. The integration of this structural computation of the objects (performed by the right hemisphere) with their functional properties and meaning would be a successive stage supported preeminently by the left hemisphere.

Prosopagnosia

Prosopagnosia (PA) is that form of VA indicating a specific deficit for the visual recognition of faces. To diagnose PA, it is necessary to exclude that a more elementary visual and perceptive dysfunction may be the cause. Patients with PA do not visually recognize the physiognomy and identity of the faces, although they can correctly identify people by the voice, emotional expressions or gait cadence. As for VA, it is possible to distinguish an apperceptive (apPA) and an associative form (AsPA) of PA.

According to the most influential cognitive model of Bruce and Young [25], which attributed to the system of face recognition specificity and sequential modularity, 2 stages are defined. The first process (dysfunctioning with apPA) analyzes the perceptive and non-emotional elemental features of the face to construct a code prototype, which, if it has already been stored in memory, provides a feeling of familiarity. Subsequently, the information progresses to identity nodes to activate, if the face is known, the memory store that contains all the semantic characteristics of that specific individual. Another distinct module is activated sequentially only from the identity nodes to match the face to its identity and relative proper name. In the case of the asPA, the processes of the first stages are adequate, but the access to the semantic information is limited.

PA behaviors manifest usually after bilateral ventral temporal lesions, generally together with other forms of VA, topographical disorientation (TD), achromatopsia, memory deficits, and visual field defects. However, clinical studies of stroke patients clearly indicated that a right lesion of the temporal-occipital associative areas is sufficient for the syndrome to emerge [26]. The specific association of face recognition abilities with the right hemisphere is supported also by functional imagery studies on normal subjects [27]. Such researches found that a restricted area (within the fusiform gyrus), "the fusiform area for faces", responds specifically to faces and not to objects, and more exactly to identity than expression [28].

Cases of developmental PA are quite rare. However, they have been always linked to abnormalities of the right posterior fusiform area [29, 30].

Compensatory training for PA, such as verbalizing distinctive facial features, could be useful in rehabilitation settings [31].

Topographical Disorientation

TD refers to the difficulty of traveling or "navigating" in a spatial environment. This syndrome should not be explained by primary visuoperceptual deficits or dementia and should be differentiated by conditions of altered perception of distances, USN, and simultagnosia.

All patients with TD show their difficulties when they have to learn the spatial configuration of a new place in which they have to move. To counteract their deficits, they try to use verbal descriptions to decompose the view in linear sequences, a strategy of the left hemisphere. The assessment of TD could be difficult but, recently, in order to standardize it, virtual reality experiences have been built. TD could be further separated in the perceptive (peDT) and mnesic (mnDT) variants. With peDT (also defined as topographic agnosia), the visual analysis of places, landmarks, and directions are primarily defective while, in the case of mnDT (also defined as topographic amnesia) the patient is not able to recollect the topographical information of the time before stroke. Another classification [32], which finds support in neuroimaging studies of normal subjects, suggests the existence of the following subtypes: landmark agnosia (impairment of using salient features/landmarks for direction), heading disorientation (impaired use of landmarks), egocentric disorientation (impaired representation of object location in comparison to the self-location), and anterograde disorientation (impairment in creating new space and environment representations).

Studies on brain-damaged patients [33] and normal subjects indicated that the right hippocampus and the right inferotemporal region are dominant for the spatial navigation (route learning, integrated representation of places, and their spatial relationships) and that this navigational network might be composed of specialized modules. The right hippocampus would be implicated in spatial memory processes on larger scales, while the right parietal lobe would calculate spatial ego or allocentric references with the aim of providing a mental map which is continuously upgraded online according to the movements of the subject. Other brain regions which are involved in spatial navigation are those of the vestibular system, the anterior and posterior cingular gyrus, the caudal nucleus, the cerebellum, the prefrontal regions, splenium, and cuneus [34].

Rehabilitation of TD could be difficult. However, functional improvement could be attained with the use of smartphone applications [35].

Dysprosody

The prosody is a communicative linguistic function, which results from the intonation, cadence, accent, and physical duration of the words. The prosody enhances the comprehension or the composed words, the basic emotions (rage, fear, sadness, surprise, disgust, pleasure), the subtle emotional aspects of the discourse (irony, sarcasm, deception, boredom, solace), and allows the differentiation of declarative, interrogative, and imperative phrases.

Thus, the expressive (affective) dysprosody is a suprasegmental deficit of language which should not be explained by a motor (dysarthria) or premotor (language apraxia) deficit, nor phonological or aphasic dysfunction (such as agrammatism and anomia). The patients with receptive dysprosody do not understand the emotional information of the phrases or the meaning of gesticulation.

Affective dysprosody could be an early predictor of post-stroke depression [36].

Several studies on brain-damaged patients [37, 38] and normal subjects demonstrated the dominant role of the right hemisphere for prosody. In acute stroke settings, the assessment of dysprosody by bedside tests could help in localizing the lesion to the right hemisphere [38]. Dysprosody, during epileptic seizures, has been linked to right hemisphere foci [39].

The profile of anatomical correlation of prosodic syndromes (motor aprosodia for anterior and receptive dysprosody for posterior lesions) seems to parallel one of the aphasic syndromes of the left hemisphere.

Functional neuroimaging studies on normal subjects also provided a dichotomous scenario for linguistic functions such as the left hemisphere dominance for phonological and phonetic aspects versus the right hemisphere dominance for the emotional aspects [40–42]. Finally, the left hemisphere seems to be involved in linguistic features on short times (at level of letters and syllables), while the right hemisphere seems to process longer intervals (at the level of words and phrases).

Dysprosody might be amenable to behavioral treatments [43].

Anosognosia

We can distinguish 2 variants of anosognosia. The first is a sensorial form, which manifests after right hemisphere damage, corresponding to the anosognosia for a specific neurologic deficit (i.e., anosognosia for hemiplegia or hemianopia), while the second is a more general disorder of not acknowledging the suitability of his own behavior to a situation or a person, a condition which is more general (resulting from "frontal" dysfunction) and is not specific to the right hemisphere damage.

The "right hemisphere anosognosia" and related phenomena (asomatognosia, somatoparaphrenia, pseudopolymyelia, anosodiaphoria, and misoplegia) are covered in detail in other sections of this book.

We emphasize the fact that anosognosia for hemiplegia manifests in its flamboyant forms in the acute phase of stroke, as it improves in shorter times, generally more rapidly than spatial neglect to which it usually associates.

It is difficult to explain anosognosia of the right hemisphere and all its related phenomena with a unitary mechanism. The transitory improvement of anosognosia with caloric vestibular stimulation, a situation which points to a mechanism of altered body schema coordinates would not explain the nature of confabulations. Furthermore, confabulations themselves could correspond to the inability of inhibiting correct responses or to a right-left hemisphere disconnection.

Finally, the large variety of the phenomena associated with anosognosia (visuoperceptive and motor deficits, spatial neglect, body schema distortions, confabulations) together with multiple lesion localizations suggests the existence, for self-body awareness, of a diffuse neuronal network for which the right hemisphere is dominant. It is important to emphasize that this network should directly intervene in almost every aspect of the conscious and unconscious self.

Misidentification Syndromes

They are rare neurologic syndromes in which the patient attributes with certainty a wrong identity (a sort of hypo-identification) to people (Capgras syndrome or doubles' illusion), to places (reduplicative amnesia), or believes that the physical appearance of a person changed into that of another (Fregoli syndrome), this last condition corresponds to a sort of hyper-identification. A parallelism can be traced between the Capgras syndrome and somatoparaphrenia (another right hemisphere syndrome). The patient with somatoparaphrenia believes that his or her paralyzed left arm belongs to another person.

In the case of intermetamorphosis, the patient believes that persons, animals or objects exchange their respective identities, while in the case of para prosopagnosia the face or a body of a known person transforms in a grotesque way (monster, vampire, lycanthrope). A delusional hermaphroditism has also been described [44]. More types of misidentification can even coexist in the same patient.

All these conditions lie at the interface between neurology and psychiatry as they can manifest either with neurologic disease (stroke, subdural hematoma, Alzheimer's disease, Lewy-body disease, drug intoxication, brain trauma, Parkinson's disease, Fahr' disease, levodopa-induced psychosis) or psychiatric disease without brain lesions (such as paranoia, schizophrenia, mania, and dissociative disorders).

Capgras syndrome and reduplicative amnesia manifest after frontal parietal, occipito-parietal, and thalamic lesions. The neural mechanisms underlying the dissociation between appearance and identity of the bodies remain speculative. However, it points to the existence of different cognitive and emotional networks for recognition (or memory) of faces and bodies, networks having different neural substrates or hemispheric dominance [45].

Mania

This syndrome manifests so rarely with stroke (less than 100 case reports) that epidemiology, clinical features, and prognostic factors are difficult to define. A new onset manic syndrome in an individual older than 40 years (more than he or she is expected for primary mania), especially when associated to other neurological signs, should point to stroke, neoplasms or frontotemporal dementia [46, 47]. Most of these cases are consequent to the damage of the right hemisphere, more specifically a ventral limbic circuit including the right orbitofrontal, prefrontal and basal temporal cortices, the dorsomedial thalamic nucleus, and the head of the caudate nucleus. Neuroleptics, mood stabilizers, lithium (its use is controversial in case of brain lesions), and benzodiazepines are possible pharmacological interventions.

A less invalidating variant is the "Gourmand syndrome" with which patients manifest a subtle obsession for fine foods, a syndrome that emerged after anterior lesions of the right hemisphere [48].

The theoretical mechanism for all the cases of secondary mania is the loss of a regulatory prefrontal control on limbic structures [49].

Conclusions

The studies of the right hemisphere syndromes suggest that this hemisphere is dominant for the physical and emotional dimensions of the human being, which are necessary for self-body-environment awareness and recognition.

Right hemisphere lesions modify the perception of space (spatial neglect, VAs, TD), of the body schema and self-awareness (anosognosia, somatoparaphrenia), can deeply disturb the expression or the emotional comprehension (dysprosody), dissociate the integration of emotional valences with identities (misidentification syndromes) and impulse control. These changes are amplified by the depletion of the attentional resources for which the right hemisphere is dominant, a phenomenon that gives to the patient the appearance of an individual less vital and less connected to the world. Finally, the right hemisphere provides a more perceptive and emotional consciousness to be integrated with the more analytical and linguistic processes of the left hemisphere.

The great mysteries of the right brain hemisphere concern the origin of the emotional sphere, the integration of the sensory with the cognitive sphere, the human consciousness, and, finally the human nature itself. Patients with brain hemisphere damage, especially in the acute phase, might appear to be in an alien world with disturbed spatial, sensory, and emotional coordinates.

The right hemisphere mysteries will be progressively revealed only by integrating the researches of different scientific disciplines (neurology, cognitive psychology, neuropsychiatry, functional neuroimaging, and neurophysiology).

Further Reading

Barton JJS, Corrow SL: Selectivity in acquired prosopagnosia: The segregation of divergent and convergent operations. Neuropsychologia 2016;83:76–87.

tom limb. In a recent systematic review concerning spinal cord stimulation, 7 out of 12 studies showed clinically significant results for pain relief [26].

The mirror therapy, aiming to produce an illusion of a whole body scheme despite the limb loss, was introduced by Ramachandran [27]. A patient, when observing his existing extremities in a mirror box, tricks his mind and introduces false messages on the existence of the amputated limb, thus diminishing pain symptoms. This method is safe, economical, and easy-to-use. It seems that patients who are not using prosthesis had greater benefit from mirror therapy. Rehabilitation for phantom limb pain using a combined procedure of mirror therapy and transcranial direct current stimulation has been proposed [28].

Immersive virtual reality has also been proposed. The patient is immersed in virtual reality and begins to percept a virtual complete body, which leads the phantom pain to deteriorate [29]. For Ortiz-Catalan et al. [30], promotion of phantom motor execution aided by machine learning, augmented and virtual reality, and gaming is a non-invasive, non-pharmacologic, and engaging treatment with no identified side-effects.

Supernumerary Phantom Limb

The supernumerary phantom limb phenomenon is a subjective sensation of the presence of a non-existent limb in addition to the regular set of 2 upper limbs and 2 lower limbs. Unlike the phantom limb of an amputee, the perception of a supernumerary limb is rarely painful.

A psychological origin for the perception of phantom supernumerary limbs was first proposed, but numerous cases occurred with normal cognitive function and without clinically detectable psychiatric illness, which suggests an organic cause.

Supernumerary phantom limbs were first reported in patients with parietal lobe lesions [31]. However, it became clear that disruption of any of the anatomical structures involved in body awareness may result in the perception of supernumerary limbs. These structures, usually involved in stroke, include the thalamus, supplementary motor area, motor cortex, posterior limb of internal capsule or pons [32–35]. Supernumerary phantom limb may be a rare symptom of epileptic seizures [36]. Some lesions are more rarely implicated in the pathogenesis of supernumerary phantom limb, such as the spinal cord injury [37] or acute inflammatory demyelinating polyneuropathy [38].

The pathogenesis of supernumerary phantom limb is not clearly defined. Different neural mechanisms have been proposed. The conventional concept emphasizes dissociation between the previously established sensorimotor representations and the lesion-induced change in communication between the cortex and the paralyzed limb. A deficit in the representation of space or disordered reality-testing abilities [39] has also been proposed for the supernumerary phantom limb. Sensory deafferentation seems to be the main mechanism in some patients. A patient reported having 2 phantom supernumerary canine teeth that pressed on her tongue after resection of hypertrophic gums [40].

Only a few data related to functional magnetic resonance imaging are available. The findings demonstrate that intentional movements of a seen and felt supernumerary phantom limb activate premotor and motor areas together with visual and sensory cortex, confirming its multimodal dimension [41]. A recent study confirmed that virtual visual feedback reduces supernumerary phantom limb phenomena [42].

Apotemnophilia

Apotemnophilia is a rare condition in which persons report an intensive desire to have one or more of their healthy limbs amputated. This disorder was named after the Greek words "apo" (away from), "temno" (piece cut off) and "philia" (love), leading to a general meaning of "love for amputation" [43].

In the first report of 2 cases by Money et al. [43] in 1977, this disorder was diagnosed as paraphilia. According to this view, following published studies linked the desire for amputation to a sexual disturbance, attributing its origin to a paraphilic disorder. Some key features were identified: male predominance, a most frequent desire of left-sided amputations, and a preference toward amputation of the leg versus the arm [44].

In 2005, First suggested that apotemnophilia may be conceptualized as an unusual dysfunction in the development of one's fundamental sense of anatomical body identity [44]. The condition was progressively named body integrity identity disorder in which persons report an intensive desire to have one or more of their healthy limbs amputated [45, 46]. This disorder can be seen as a mismatch between the mental body image and the physical body shape, influencing the lives of affected persons in an extreme way [44, 46]. Next to the wish for limb amputation, a variant body integrity identity disorder was reported: the desire for non-functioning limbs, which concerned mainly females [46, 47].

In the last decade, the body integrity identity disorder evolved from a psychological to a neurological syndrome. Based on similarities with neurological symptoms (asomatognosia, somatoparaphrenia, misoplegia) associated with damage to right parietal cortex, some authors have mentioned possible neurological causes for the desire for limb amputation [44, 48]. The inadequate activation of the right superior parietal lobule leads to the unnatural situation in which the sufferers can feel the limb in question being touched without it actually incorporating into their body image, with a resulting desire for amputation. The term xenomelia was introduced as a more appropriate name than apotemnophilia or body integrity identity disorder, for this right parietal lobe syndrome [49, 50].

Conclusion

A functional magnetic resonance imaging study suggests that altered somatosensory processing in the premotor cortex is associated with the feeling of lack of ownership in body integrity identity disorder, which may be related to altered integration of somatosensory and proprioceptive information [51]. A recent magnetic resonance imaging study using voxel-based morphometry suggests that body integrity identity disorder is associated with structural brain anomalies. It showed a reduced grey matter volume in the left dorsal and ventral premotor cortices, and larger grey matter volume in the cerebellum. These regions are thought to be crucial for the experience of body-ownership and the integration of multisensory information [52].

To date, there is no effective treatment available for body identity disorder. Consequently, patients resort to self-amputation because they are not able to enlist a surgeon to amputate their healthy limb. Self-amputation reveals a 100% satisfaction rate. Patients report a better quality of life; they do not desire any additional amputations, nor do they regret their decision [46]. Nevertheless self-amputation leads to complications and sometimes death. In some cases, authors offer arguments in favor of elective surgical amputation that can prevent complications and death in patients who are contemplating self-amputation [53].

References

1 Nikolajsen L, Jensen TS: Phantom limb pain. Br J Anaesth 2001;87:107–116.

2 Trevelyan EG, Turner WA, Robinson N: Perceptions of phantom limb pain in lower limb amputees and its effect on quality of life: a qualitative study. Br J Pain 2016;10:70–77.

3 Ramachandran VS, Hirstein W: The perception of phantom limbs. The D.O. Hebb lecture. Brain 1998; 121:1603–1630.

4 Hunter JP, Katz J, Davis KD: Dissociation of phantom limb phenomena from stump tactile spatial acuity and sensory thresholds. Brain 2004;128:308–320.

5 Tatu L, Bogousslavsky J, Boller F: Phantoms in artists: the lost limbs of Blaise Cendrars, Arthur Rimbaud and Paul Wittgenstein. J Hist Neurosci 2014; 23:355–366.

6 Giummarra MJ, Moseley GL: Phantom limb pain and bodily awareness: current concepts and future directions. Curr Opin Anaesthesiol 2011;24:524–531.

7 Katz J, Melzack R: Pain "memories" in phantom limbs: review and clinical observations. Pain 1990; 43:319–336.

8 Paré A: De la manière de traiter les plaies faites par harquebuse. Paris, Arnoult l'Angelié, 1582.

9 Descartes R: Les Méditations de René Descartes Touchant La Première Philosophie. 6e Meditation, ed 2. Paris, Henry Le Gras,1690.

10 Porterfield W: A Treatise On the Eye: the Manner and Phenomena of Vision. vol 1. Edinburgh, Hamilton and Balfour, 1759.

11 Bell C: The Nervous System of the Human Body. London, Longman, 1830.

12 Mitchell SW: The case of George Dedlow. Atlantic Monthly 1866;XVIII(105):1–11.

13 Mitchell SW: Phantom limbs. Lippincott Magazine 1871;8:563–569.

14 Mitchell SW: Injuries of Nerves and their Consequences. Philadelphia, Lippincott, 1872.

15 Tatu L: The missing hands of Blaise Cendrars in: Neurological Disorders in Famous Artists – Part 3. Basel, Karger, 2010, pp 143–159.

16 MacIver K, Lloyd DM, Kelly S, Roberts N, Nurmikko T: Phantom limb pain, cortical reorganization and the therapeutic effect of mental imagery. Brain 2008; 131:2181–2191.

17 Simoes EL, Bramati I, Rodrigues E, Franzoi A, Moll J, Lent R, et al: Functional expansion of sensorimotor representation and structural reorganization of callosal connections in lower limb amputees. J Neurosci 2012;32:3211–3220.

18 Raffin E, Giraux P, Reilly KT: The moving phantom: motor execution or motor imagery? Cortex 2012;48: 746–757.

19 Flor H, Elbert T, Knecht S, Wienbruch C, Pantev C, Birbaumer N, et al: Phantom-limb pain as a perceptual correlate of cortical reorganization following arm amputation. Nature 1995;375:482–484.

20 Makin TR, Scholz J, Filippini N, Henderson Slater D, Tracey I, Johansen-Berg H: Phantom pain is associated with preserved structure and function in the former hand area. Nat Commun 2013;4:1570.

21 Boström KJ, de Lussanet MH, Weiss T, Puta C, Wagner H: A computational model unifies apparently contradictory findings concerning phantom pain. Sci Rep 2014;4:5298.

22 Raffin E, Richard N, Giraux P, Reilly KT: Primary motor cortex changes after amputation correlate with phantom limb pain and the ability to move the phantom limb. Neuroimage 2016;130:134–144.
23 Alviar MJM, Hale T, Dungca M: Pharmacologic interventions for treating phantom limb pain; in: Alviar MJ, (ed) Cochrane Database of Systematic Reviews. Chichester, John Wiley & Sons, 2016.
24 Trevelyan EG, Turner WA, Summerfield-Mann L, Robinson N: Acupuncture for the treatment of phantom limb syndrome in lower limb amputees: a randomised controlled feasibility study. Trials 2016; 17:519.
25 Malavera A, Silva FA, Fregni F, Carrillo S, Garcia RG: Repetitive transcranial magnetic stimulation for phantom limb pain in land mine victims: a double-blinded, randomized, sham-controlled trial. J Pain 2016;17:911–918.
26 Aiyer R, Barkin RL, Bhatia A, Gungor S: A systematic review on the treatment of phantom limb pain with spinal cord stimulation. Pain Manag 2017;7: 59–69.
27 Guenther K: '"It's all done with mirrors": V.S. Ramachandran and the material culture of phantom limb research. Med Hist 2016;60:342–358.
28 Pinto CB, Saleh Velez FG, Bolognini N, Crandell D, Merabet LB, Fregni F: Optimizing rehabilitation for phantom limb pain using mirror therapy and transcranial direct current stimulation: a randomized, double-blind clinical trial study protocol. JMIR Res Protoc 2016;5:e138.
29 Osumi M, Ichinose A, Sumitani M, Wake N, Sano Y, Yozu A, et al: Restoring movement representation and alleviating phantom limb pain through short-term neurorehabilitation with a virtual reality system. Eur J Pain 2017;21:140–147.
30 Ortiz-Catalan M, Guðmundsdóttir RA, Kristoffersen MB, Zepeda-Echavarria A, Caine-Winterberger K, Kulbacka-Ortiz K, et al: Phantom motor execution facilitated by machine learning and augmented reality as treatment for phantom limb pain: a single group, clinical trial in patients with chronic intractable phantom limb pain. Lancet 2016;388:2885–2894.
31 Critchley M: The Parietal Lobes. New York, Hafner, 1953.
32 Miyazawa N, Hayashi M, Komiya K, Akiyama I: Supernumerary phantom limbs associated with left hemispheric stroke: case report and review of the literature. Neurosurgery 2004;54:228–231; discussion 231.
33 Canavero S, Bonicalzi V, Castellano G, Perozzo P, Massa-Micon B: Painful supernumerary phantom arm following motor cortex stimulation for central poststroke pain. Case report. J Neurosurg 1999;91: 121–123.
34 Staub F, Bogousslavsky J, Maeder P, Maeder-Ingvar M, Fornari E, Ghika J, et al: Intentional motor phantom limb syndrome. Neurology 2006;67:2140–2146.
35 Yoo SD, Kim DH, Jeong YS, Chon J, Bark J: Atypical supernumerary phantom limb and phantom limb pain in two patients with pontine hemorrhage. J Korean Med Sci 2011;26:844.
36 Millonig A, Bodner T, Donnemiller E, Wolf E, Unterberger I: Supernumerary phantom limb as a rare symptom of epileptic seizures – case report and literature review. Epilepsia 2011;52:e97–e100.
37 Curt A, Yengue CN, Hilti LM, Brugger P: Supernumerary phantom limbs in spinal cord injury. Spinal Cord 2011;49:588–595.
38 Melinyshyn AN, Gofton TE, Schulz V: Supernumerary phantom limbs in ICU patients with acute inflammatory demyelinating polyneuropathy. Neurology 2016;86:1726–1728.
39 Sellal F, Renaseau-leclerc C, Labrecque R: [The man with 6 arms. An analysis of supernumerary phantom limbs after right hemisphere stroke]. Rev Neurol (Paris) 1996;152:190–195.
40 Jacome DE: Case report Dracula's teeth syndrome. Headache 2001;41:892–894.
41 Khateb A, Simon SR, Dieguez S, Lazeyras F, Momjian-Mayor I, Blanke O, et al: Seeing the phantom: A functional magnetic resonance imaging study of a supernumerary phantom limb. Ann Neurol 2009;65: 698–705.
42 Katayama O, Iki H, Sawa S, Osumi M, Morioka S: The effect of virtual visual feedback on supernumerary phantom limb pain in a patient with high cervical cord injury: a single-case design study. Neurocase 2015;21:786–792.
43 Money J, Jobaris R, Furth G: Apotemnophilia: two cases of self demand amputation as paraphilia. J Sex Res 1977;43:115–125.
44 First MB: Desire for amputation of a limb: paraphilia, psychosis, or a new type of identity disorder. Psychol Med 2005;35:919–928.
45 Brugger P, Lenggenhager B: The bodily self and its disorders: neurological, psychological and social aspects. Curr Opin Neurol 2014;27:644–652.
46 Blom RM, Hennekam RC, Denys D: Body integrity identity disorder. PLoS One 2012;7:e34702.
47 Giummarra MJ, Bradshaw JL, Hilti LM, Nicholls ME, Brugger P: Paralyzed by desire: a new type of body integrity identity disorder. Cogn Behav Neurol 2012;25:34–41.
48 Brang D, McGeoch PD, Ramachandran VS: Apotemnophilia: a neurological disorder. Neuroreport 2008;19:1305–1306.
49 McGeoch PD, Brang D, Song T, Lee RR, Huang M, Ramachandran VS: Xenomelia: a new right parietal lobe syndrome. J Neurol Neurosurg Psychiatry 2011; 82:1314–1319.

50 Sedda A, Bottini G: Apotemnophilia, body integrity identity disorder or xenomelia? Psychiatric and neurologic etiologies face each other. Neuropsychiatr Dis Treat 2014;10:1255.
51 van Dijk MT, van Wingen GA, van Lammeren A, Blom RM, de Kwaasteniet BP, Scholte HS, et al: Neural basis of limb ownership in individuals with body integrity identity disorder. PLoS One 2013;8:e72212.
52 Blom R, Vulink NC, van der Wal SJ, Nakamae T, Tan Z, Derks EM, et al: Body integrity identity disorder crosses culture: case reports in the Japanese and Chinese literature. Neuropsychiatr Dis Treat 2016;12: 1419.
53 White A: Body integrity identity disorder beyond amputation: consent and liberty. HEC Forum 2014; 26:225–236.

Prof. Laurent Tatu
Department of Neuromuscular Diseases and Department of Anatomy
CHRU Besançon, University of Franche-Comté
3 boulevard Fleming
FR–25000 Besançon (France)
E-Mail laurent.tatu@univ-fcomte.fr

Bogousslavsky J (ed): Neurologic-Psychiatric Syndromes in Focus. Part I – From Neurology to Psychiatry.
Front Neurol Neurosci. Basel, Karger, 2018, vol 41, pp 23–27 (DOI: 10.1159/000475689)

Misoplegia

Montserrat G. Delgado[a] • Julien Bogousslavsky[b]

[a]Neurology Service, Hospital Universitario Central de Asturias, Oviedo, Spain; [b]Neurocenter, Swiss Medical Network, Clinique Valmont, Glion/Montreux, Switzerland

Abstract

In 1974, Critchley described misoplegia as the phenomenon in which a hemiplegic patient develops a morbid dislike towards the offending immobile limbs. Patients with misoplegia may employ, but more commonly strike their paretic limbs not recognized as self. The pathophysiological mechanism is not well understood. The handful of cases of misoplegia described in the literature, frequently presented a right hemispheric damage. However, patients with chronic spinal cord injury may also present this symptomatology. Not only the modification of behavior by this organic injury, but also the patient reaction to disability and previous personality, may provoke the emergence of misoplegia, probably from other right hemispheric self unawareness syndromes. No data exists related to treatment option, but we have to remember that the lack of awareness of the deficits in these patients makes the rehabilitation process difficult. Misoplegia is one of the passionate syndromes of the still "not-enough well-known" self-awareness syndromes of the right hemisphere, which shows how brain damage goes much further beyond neurological deficit.

Introduction

Regions in the brain exist whose affectation can give symptomatology that could be confused with psychiatric pathology. Among these, the parietal lobe gives a characteristic symptomatology constituting one of the better known pathologies in the field of body awareness disease [1].

In 1914, Babinski noted the lack of consciousness of the hemiplegics patients of their neurological deficit (anosognosia) [2], mainly in right lobe lesions but also in left

Diagnosis

Diagnosis remains clinical. Critchley described misoplegia as a critical attitude in hemiplegic patients with right hemispheric lesions [6]. From mildly paranoid reaction to frankly psychotic types of thinking and behavior may insidiously develop, and the patient may violently strike the affecting limb [6]. Commonly, misoplegia includes physical acts such as striking and beating the hemiplegic extremity (misoplegia in the highest degree) [6, 9]. We have also seen a patient who squashed burning cigarettes on her arm, sometimes considering her paralyzed limb as baby doll and talking to it with promises of future punishment, while also occasionally cajoling it with her good arm.

Misoplegia was also reported in a 10-year-old child by Moss et al. [16]. The authors described 2 differential characteristics regarding misoplegia in adults: the desire for the limbs to be replaced and the coexistence of anosognosia and misoplegia [16]. As mentioned previously, patients with chronic spinal cord injury may present misoplegia [15].

After reviewing the literature, we have noted that misoplegia is a rare entity, and only a handful of cases have been described. This is in part due to the complexity of the right hemisphere in self-awareness, with a diverse symptomatology and multiple combinations [17]. Thus, a misdiagnosis of misoplegia is possible due to an overlapping with other well-known right hemisphere symptoms, making possible a broad range of neurological symptoms [10].

Treatment and Management

No data exist about the treatment and management of misoplegia. In the first descriptions, Critchley supported that a change in attitude towards anosognosia is in part, due to the intervention of nurses in attendance, visiting relatives, and the doctor in charge of the case [6].

Psychoanalytic methods suggested that anosognosia and misoplegia share a common unconscious route [12, 14], and some studies have shown that symptoms from right hemisphere damage such as neglect and anosognosia can temporarily be alleviated using this method [17]. Psychotherapeutic interviews in these patients could make them temporarily aware of their deficit [12, 14]. When paralysis was recognized, all the patients showed signs of depression [12, 14]. However, there are no reports about the use of anti-depressive treatment in these patients.

The Neuropsychoanalytic Study Group, Frankfurt/Cologne has performed psychoanalytic therapy with a group of patients with right hemispheric lesions presenting neglect/anosognosia [17]. The results of the study indicated that defense against depression is not the only cause of the syndrome [17]. A failure to construct a body schema, as a result of the paralyzed side of the body no longer being represented, is also involved [17]. In this sense, some authors suggested that treatments addressed to increase the function of right hemisphere networks, supporting agency and body ownership, may promise reduce in certain types of self-injurious acts [13].

In spite of this, it has to be remembered that the lack of awareness of deficits in these patients make the rehabilitation process difficult. In this way, the presence of anosognosia has been described as an extremely powerful predictor of poor outcome after stroke [12].

Conclusions

Misoplegia is one of the passionate syndromes of the still "not-enough well-known" self-awareness syndromes of the right hemisphere, which shows how brain damage goes much further beyond neurological deficit.

References

1 Critchley M: Psychiatric symptoms and parietal disease: differential diagnosis. Proc R Soc Med 1964;57:422–428.

2 Babinski J: Contribution à l'étude des troubles mentaux dans l'hémiplégie organique cérébrale (anosognosie). Rev Neurologique 1914;27:845–848.

3 Critchley M: Personification of paralysed limbs in hemiplegics. Br Med J 1955;30:284–286.

4 Critchley M: Observations on anosodiaphoria. Encéphale 1957;46:540–546.

5 Bogousslavsky J, Kumral E, Regli F, Assal G, Ghika J: Acute hemiconcern: a right anterior parietotemporal syndrome. J Neurol Neurosurg Psychiatry 1995;58:428–432.

6 Critchley M: Misoplegia, or hatred of hemiplegia. Mt Sinai J Med 1974;41:82–87.

7 Pearce JM: Misoplegia. Eur Neurol 2007;57:62–64.

8 Critchley M, Russell WR, Zangwill OL: Discussion on parietal lobe syndromes. Proc R Soc Med 1951;44:337–346.

9 Baier B, Karnath HO: Tight link between our sense of limb ownership and self-awareness of actions. Stroke 2008;39:486–488.

10 Loetscher T, Regard M, Brugger P: Misoplegia: a review of the literature and a case without hemiplegia. J Neurol Neurosurg Psychiatry 2006;77:1099–1100.

11 Schwartz RL, Barrett AM, Kim M, Heilman KM: Ipsilesional intentional neglect and the effect of cueing. Neurology 1999;53:2017–2022.

12 Turnbull OH, Jones K, Reed-Screen J: Implicit awareness of deficit in anosognosia? An emotion-based account of denial of deficit. Neuropsychoanalysis 2002;4:69–87.

13 Borah S, McConnell B, Hughes R, Kluger B: Potential relationship of self-injurious behavior to right temporo-parietal lesions. Neurocase 2016;22:269–272.

14 Kaplan-Solms KL, Solms M: Clinical studies in neuropsychoanalysis: Introduction of a depth neuropsychology. London, Karnac Books, 2000, pp 148–199.

15 Scandola M, Aglioti SM, Avesani R, Bertagnoni G, Marangoni A, Moro V: Corporeal illusions in chronic spinal cord injuries. Conscious Cogn 2017;49:278–290.

16 Moss AD, Turnbull OH: Hatred of the hemiparetic limbs (misoplegia) in a 10 year old child. J Neurol Neurosurg Psychiatry 1996;61:210.

17 Röckerath K: Neglect and anosognosia. A challenge for psychoanalysis. Psychoanalytic treatment of neurological patients with hemi-neglect. Psychoanalytische Perspectieven 2002;4:611–631.

Montserrat G. Delgado, MD
Hospital Universitario Central de Asturias
Plaza Fernando Álvarez, número 1, 6° H.
33006 Oviedo (Spain)
E-Mail mglezdelgado@yahoo.es

Bogousslavsky J (ed): Neurologic-Psychiatric Syndromes in Focus. Part I – From Neurology to Psychiatry.
Front Neurol Neurosci. Basel, Karger, 2018, vol 41, pp 28–39 (DOI: 10.1159/000475692)

Pali and Echo Phenomena: Symptoms of Persistence and Perseveration

Eloi Magnin[a–c] · Elisabeth Medeiros de Bustos[b, c] · Thierry Moulin[b, c]

[a]Memory Research and Resource Center (Centre Mémoire Ressources et Recherche – CMRR), Department of Neurology, Besançon University Hospital, [b]Clinical and Integrative Neuroscience, Research Laboratory 481, Bourgogne Franche-Comté University, and [c]Department of Neurology, Besançon University Hospital, Besançon, France

Abstract

Some neurological or psychiatric positive, productive symptoms are an abnormal persistence of a sensorial feeling or abnormal repetition of a motor, behavioral or cognitive process corresponding to a perseverative symptom. Palinopsia, palinacousis, and related sensorial symptoms have been described. Verbal and motor symptoms include echolalia, palilalia, echopraxia, and motor perseveration. Cognitive disorders induce perseverative behavior, perseverative thinking, including palipsychism, flashbulb memories, and reduplicative paramnesia (also known as "palimnesia") and many related perseverative symptoms. We propose a review of physiological phenomena and pathological symptoms involving these perseverative or repetitive characteristics and discuss the potential mechanisms and neural network involved in this productive semiology.

Introduction

Palin is a Greek word, meaning "again" or "anew" and *echo* means "a repetition of sound," and was also a mythological cursed nymph presenting mutism, echolalia, and palilalia (Fig. 1). Some neurological or psychiatric positive symptoms are abnormal persistence of a sensorial feeling or abnormal repetition of a behavior corresponding to a perseverative symptom. We will describe, according to each sensorial, motor or cognitive modality, some of these phenomena involving perseverative or repetitive features from normal physiological phenomena observed in healthy subjects to abnormal symptoms observed during pathological situations. Then, the underlying mechanisms and neural network involved in these phenomena will be discussed.

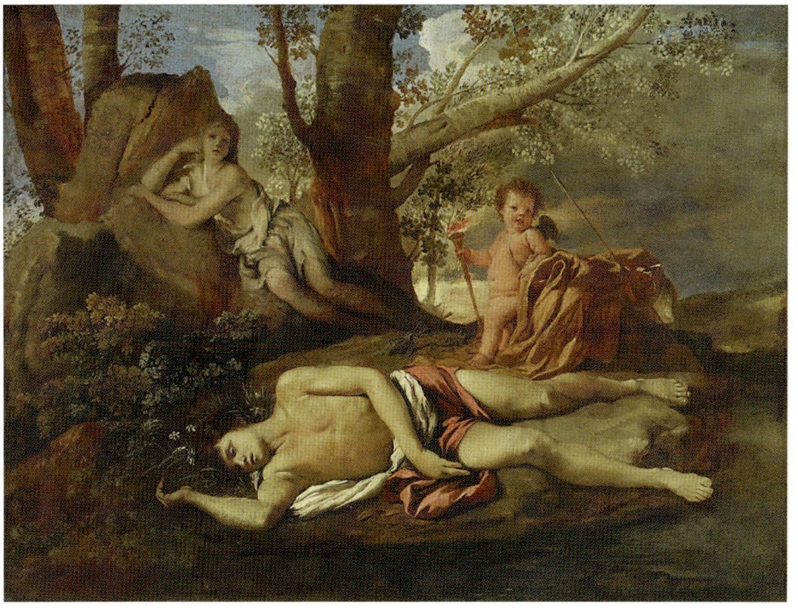

Fig. 1. Echo et Narcisse by Nicolas Poussin (about 1630; Louvre Museum, France). Both these mythical characters presented repetitive and perseverative disorders after God's curses. Echo, a talkative nymph, presented mutism with the exception of an echolalia-palilia after Juno's curse. Narcissus, a proud and disdainful man, presented misidentification and preservative gazing behavior of his mirrored reflection after Nemesis' curse. Photo © Musée du Louvre, Dist. RMN-Grand Palais/Martine Beck-Coppola.

Epidemiology

Description of Pali and Echo Phenomena

Sensorial Modalities

Preservative and repetitive symptoms can occur during the treatment of sensorial stimuli. Some of these symptoms occur in healthy subjects under specific conditions, while other symptoms are associated with pathological situations. For each sensorial modality, we will report classical symptoms, and then describe some of the rare variants of those symptoms.

Visual Symptoms

Physiological Afterimages or Retinal Persistence. Retinal persistence are physiological afterimages that appear after the visual focus is shifted following a bright stimulus. These physiological images are frequently negative afterimages (i.e., opposite color to the color of the original stimulus), but sometimes briefly positive afterimages (same color) can occur after a very bright stimulus. These phenomena can be seen in the same location as the original stimulus in the visual field regardless of eye movement with either eye open, with both eyes open, or with both eyes shut, and often disappear

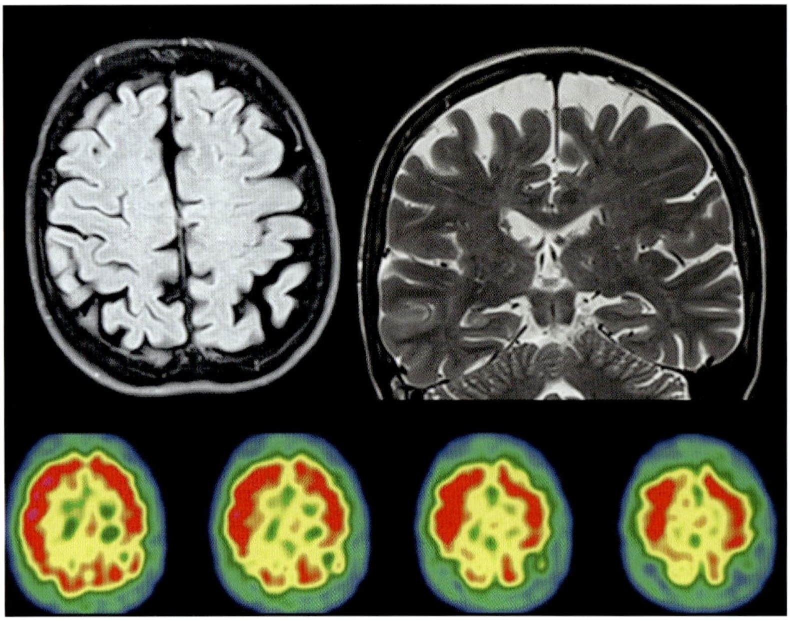

Fig. 2. MRI and cerebral perfusion (HMPAO-SPECT) showing superior temporal atrophy and hypoperfusion in a 67-year-old woman with posterior cortical atrophy syndrome presenting apraxia, labial echopraxia, and delayed palinopsia.

by blinking. Mechanisms involved in retinal persistence are thought to be due to bleaching of photochemical pigments or neural adaptation in the retina (bottom-up), but cortical involvement (top-down) is also suspected [1].

Palinopsia. Palinopsia, a rare symptom initially described during the 1960s, is the persistence or recurrence of visual images or visual perseveration after cessation of the original stimulus [2–4] (Fig. 2). Gersztenkorn and Lee [5] reviewed 128 cases of palinopsia from the literature to describe multiple types of visual symptoms and the wide variety of etiologies involved in palinopsia. Palinoptic afterimages are positive (i.e., isochromatic to the original stimulus). It can be immediate or delayed (several hours after perception). Palinopsia are mostly due to occipital disorders; sometimes parietal and rarely temporal disorders can be involved. Right-sided disorders are the most frequent cause of palinopsia, but the latter can also occur as a result of left-sided disorders. Iatrogenic origin was also reported.

Rare variants of palinoptic symptoms have been reported.

Variant of Palinoptic Symptoms and Associated Disorders

Akinetopic Palinopsia or Visual Trailing. Akinetopsia is impaired motion perception. Akinetopic palinopsia (visual trailing) is sometimes reported as stroboscopic vision. Motion appears fragmented and afterimages are left in the location where the moving object was observed [6].

Cerebral Polyopia and Entomopia. Cerebral polyopia corresponds to 2 or more duplicated images monocular bilaterally and binocularly arranged in ordered rows or columns after fixation on an object [7–9]. Palinoptic polyopia or entomopia is characterized by perseverated polyopic images that remain after perceived movement, and create hundreds of palinoptic images [10].

Visual Allesthesia. Visual allesthesia correspond to the occurrence of a duplicated image in the opposite hemifield of the original observed image [11].

Auditive Symptoms

Physiologic or Pathological "Song in the Mind." Intrusive involuntary musical imagery is also known as earworms or ohrwurms, or involuntary musical imagery [12]. It involves involuntarily recalled, short, looping fragments of melodies or lyrics or other auditive imagery that may last from minutes to hours. It can occur in the absence of neurological, psychiatric, or ear disease. It can also become a pathological musical obsession, especially in obsessive-compulsive disorders [13].

Palinacousis. Palinacousis is a rare symptom initially described in 1971 by Jacobs, Feldman, and Bender [14]. Only 21 cases are reported in the literature [14–22]. This symptom is characterized by an "echo" phenomenon, with illusory perseveration or recurrence of an auditory stimulus after cessation of the original stimulus, usually described following a left temporal lesion, frequently of tumoral or vascular origin. Seizures or postictal mechanisms are most often reported [17]. Four cases have been described concerning right-sided lesions in the median geniculate body [22] and the temporoparietal junction [23], inferior and middle temporal lesion with sparing of the superior temporal cortex [21], and right parietal hemorrhage [16] and one case with bilateral temporoparietal lesions [20]. Some cases of palinacousis are triggered by specific material, such as verbal material or music. It can be immediate or delayed (several hours after perception), and triggered regardless of the ear which perceived the stimulus, with the feeling that the echo is bilateral (i.e., in both two ears) or lateralized (i.e., only one ear).

Palinendophonia. Palinendophonia is the perseveration of "inner speech" (subvocal thoughts, silent reading) reported in association with palinacousis by Magnin et al. [21] in a case of meningoencephalitis with a right temporal lesion, with sparing of the superior temporal cortex including the Heschl gyrus and the superior temporal sulcus (Fig. 3).

Sensitive Perception

Persistence of sensitive feeling can also occur in some pathological situations.

Physiological Pain after-Sensation. Pain after-sensation is the persistence of pain after the discontinuation of nociceptive stimulus. Short pain after-sensation is a physiological phenomenon, but prolonged after-sensation can be observed during hyperpathia, hyperalgesia, or sensory over-responsivity. They are considered to be manifestations of central sensitization [24, 25].

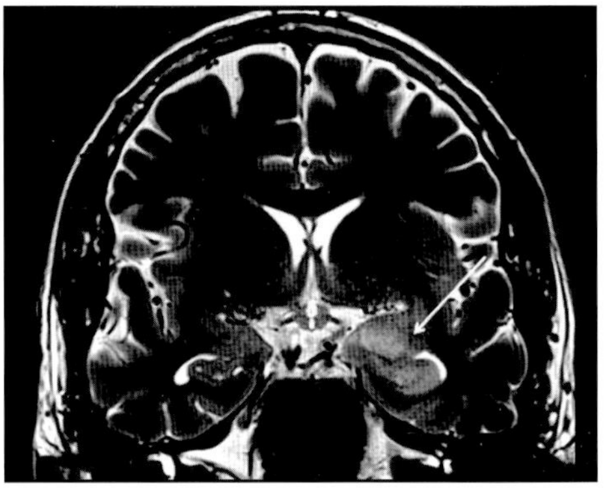

Fig. 4. MRI with left internal temporal lobe T2 hypersignal in a 58-year-old patient with a lymphoma presenting frequent episodes of flashbulb traumatic memories revealing a paraneoplasic encephalitis (personal case).

prefrontal cortex. A decrease in left DLPFC activity might induce left temporal hyperactivity, a structure associated with language and inner speech, during rumination [45, 46].

Flashbulb Memories and other Repetitive Memories
Flashbulb Memories and other Repetitive Memories. Flashbulb memories or flashbacks are vivid recollections of memory-associated emotions of event considered to be of particular significance, frequently observed during post-traumatic stress disorders but can also occur during neurological pathology [47] (Fig. 4). Other memories can spontaneously be recollected without an emotional context. Complex cases present vivid rehearsal memories (with or without emotional significance), frequently considered as hypermnesia but that can sometimes be considered to be "palimnesia."

Delusional Misidentification Syndromes
Reduplicative paramnesia is a reduplicative misidentification delusion in which a place, an object, a person, a part of the body (supernumerary phantom limbs; see Phantom Phenomena), or an event is duplicated. Doppelgänger is a kind of reduplicative paramnesia in which patients believe they have a clone or that they themselves are a clone of their own "self." The reduplicative mechanisms frequently occurred after the right hemisphere of bifrontal lesions and might involve an abnormal memory, visuospatial and conceptual integration [48].

Fregoli syndrome corresponds to a delusional misidentification syndrome, inducing the belief that a person has been replaced by another person in disguise even if their physical appearance is totally different. It can be considered as a perseverative and repetitive attribution of a defined identity to other people [49]. This hyperidentification is opposed to hypoidentification that occurs in Capgras syndrome or misidentification of reflection. Capgras syndrome is a delusion in which known persons are not identified but considered systematically as doppelganger [50]. This doppelganger attribution might also be considered as a kind of perseverative misidentification with a persistent "doppelganger" feeling.

Table 1. Citation linking memory and persistence of information

"Memory is a kind of way (or weight – whichever it should be) that the mind has got upon it, in virtue of which the sensation excited endures a little longer than the cause which excited it. There is thus induced a state of things in which mental images, and even physical sensations (if there can be such a thing as a physical sensation) exist by virtue of association, though the conditions which originally called them into existence no longer continue. This is as the echo continuing to reverberate after the sound has ceased" Samuel Butler (1835–1902), The Note-Books of Samuel Butler, 1912.

Disease Pathogenesis

Persistence, imitation, and repetition are important physiological processes during the early development of language, gesture, and social behavior. During maturation, these behaviors should be inhibited to enable contextual adapted behavior [51, 52]. Abnormal echo and pali phenomena inducing persistence, imitative and/or repetitive symptoms might provide some clues on the cognitive mechanisms involved in the normal functioning and the associated neural circuit, such as in memory or executive functions, and especially inhibition.

These phenomena might occur after a dysfunction at any stage of the information treatment pathway from the sensorial stimulus reception to signal transmission and cortical treatment of information. Abnormalities of stimuli, receptors, afferent nerves and white matter, the basal ganglia network, primary sensorial cortices and associative sensorial cortices, and frontal lobes might be involved in this semiology.

Sensorial echo and pali phenomena are on the limits of illusory and hallucinatory symptoms, suggesting dysfunction of perception or sensorial memory. Illusory symptoms corresponding to a distorted perception of a real external stimulus (i.e., prolonged stimulus with the same location and time compared to original stimulus) are related to perception disorders while hallucinatory symptoms corresponding to a generated feeling where no stimulus exists (i.e., occurs regardless of the initial location and time of the stimulus) correspond to memory disorders [5]. A recent unitary perceptual-mnemonic model linked perception and memory in the same process (Table 1) [53, 54]. Maintenance and rehearsal systems such as phonological loops, visuospatial sketchpads, episodic buffers, and mirror neurons system are involved in short-term memory and working memory [55], and play a role in many other cognitive processes [56], such as language [57], gestural treatment [58], and imagery [59]. A dysfunction of these maintenance and rehearsal processes inducing abnormal repetition of brain activation might therefore induce persistence and perseverative disorders. Different disorders might be involved in this dysregulation with bottom-up mechanisms, such as hyperintense stimulus, receptor and primary sensitive cortices hyperexcitability, especially during partial epilepsy and migraine

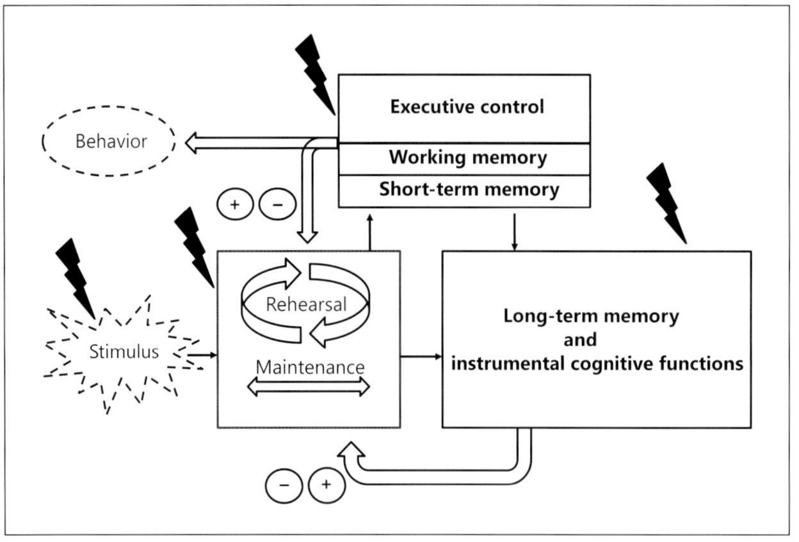

Fig. 5. Maintenance and rehearsal systems are involved in multiple cognitive processes. Many disorders occurring at different steps (black lightening) might deregulate these mechanisms and induce immediate or delayed sensitive, cognitive or behavioral pali and/or echo phenomena.

with aura, and top down mechanisms, such as hyperstimulation or hypoinhibition of executive control, memory, or instrumental cognitive functions (Fig. 5). Executive functions might have a major role in the regulation of these processes because persistent and perseverative symptoms frequently occurred after fronto-basal loop dysfunction [43].

Pharmaceutical responses give some clues about the underlying mechanisms involved in pali and echo phenomena. As several drugs inducing palinopsia affect 5-HT2 receptors (such as LSD, MDMA, nefazodone, trazodone, risperidone, zonisamide, mirtazapine, and topiramate), an increase in serotonergic activity is suspected in the pathophysiology of palinopsia [60]. Antiepileptic efficacy of these symptoms suggests potential neuronal hyperexcitability. Neuroleptic effects and antiparkinsonian drug side effects could also suggest an imbalance in the fronto-basal loop modulated by mesocorticolimbic and nigrostriatal dopaminergic pathways [42].

Conclusion

Persistent or perseverative phenomena might occur in a wide range of neurological diseases such as epilepsy, Parkinson's disease and other neurodegenerative disorders, as well as in psychiatric diseases with Gilles de la Tourette syndrome, obsessional compulsive disorders, and schizophrenia. This emphasizes the close association between the two disciplines. A better understanding of these symptoms is important for both neurologists and psychiatrists in clinical practice. Common semiology between these 2 medical specialities should also be explored using neuroscientist and neuropsychologist approaches to better understand normal and pathologic cognitive mechanisms and neural pathways involved in these persistent and perseverative symptoms.

References

1 Galifret Y: Visual persistence and cinema? C R Biol 2006;329:369–385.

2 Bender MB: Disorders in visual perception; in Halpern L (ed): Problems of Dynamic Neurology. Jerusalem, Jerusalem Post Press, 1963, pp 319–375.

3 Bender MB, Feldman M, Sobin AJ: Palinopsia. Brain 1968;91:321–338.

4 Kinsbourne M, Warrington E: A study of visual perseveration. J Neurol Neurosurg Psychiatry 1963;26: 468–475.

5 Gersztenkorn D, Lee AG: Palinopsia revamped: a systematic review of the literature. Surv Ophthalmol 2015;60:1–35.

6 Sierra-Hidalgo F, de Pablo-Fernandez E: Palinopsia induced by topiramate and zonisamide in a patient with migraine. Clin Neuropharmacol 2013;36:63–64.

7 Bender MB, Sobin AJ: Polyopia and palinopsia in homonymous fields of vision. Trans Am Neurol Assoc 1963;88:56–59.

8 Jones MR, Waggoner R, Hoyt WF: Cerebral polyopia with extrastriate quadrantanopia: report of a case with magnetic resonance documentation of V2/V3 cortical infarction. J Neuroophthalmol 1999; 19:1–6.

9 Zakaria A, Lalani I, Belorgey L, Jay Foreman P: Focal occipital seizures with cerebral polyopia. Epileptic Disord. 2006;8:295–297.

10 Lopez JR, Adornato BT, Hoyt WF: "Entomopia:" a remarkable case of cerebral polyopia. Neurology 1993;43:2145–2146.

11 Bender MB, Shapiro MF, Teuber HL: Allesthesia and disturbance of the body scheme. Arch Neurol Psychiatry 1949;62:222–235.

12 Williamson VJ, Jilka SR, Fry J, Finkel S, Müllensiefen D, Stewart L: How do "earworms" start? Classifying the everyday circumstances of involuntary musical imagery. Psychol Music 2011;40:259–284.

13 Taylor S, McKay D, Miguel EC, De Mathis MA, Andrade C, Ahuja N, Sookman D, Kwon JS, Huh MJ, Riemann BC, Cottraux J, O'Connor K, Hale LR, Abramowitz JS, Fontenelle LF, Storch EA: Musical obsessions: a comprehensive review of neglected clinical phenomena. J Anxiety Disord 2014;28:580–589.

14 Jacobs L, Feldman M, Bender MB: Palinacousis of persistent auditory sensations. Trans Am Neurol Assoc 1971;96:123–126.

15 Sánchez-Martínez A, Benito-Orejas JI, Campos-Blanco DM, Morais-Pérez D: Palinacousis secondary to brain damage from methotrexate. Acta Otorrino laringol Esp 2016;67:349–351.

16 Rosenberg D, Latorre JG: Hearing one's voice in your speech: an unusual case of palinacousis due to acute intracerebral hemorrhage. Neurologist 2016; 21:13–15.

17 Mohamed W, Ahuja N, Shah A: Palinacousis – evidence to suggest a post-ictal phenomenon. J Neurol Sci 2012;317:6–12.

18 Jacobs L, Feldman M, Bender MB: Palinacousis of persistent auditory sensations. Trans Am Neurol Assoc 1971;96:123–126.

19 Jacobs L, Feldman M, Diamond SP, Bender MB: Palinacousis: persistent or recurring auditory sensations. Cortex 1973;9:275–287.

20 Bega D, Wang N, Klein JP: Reversible palinacousis from intracranial metastases. Neuro Hospitalist 2014;4:22–25.

21 Magnin E, Ryff I, Hague S, Decavel P, Vighetto A, Moulin T: A new symptom, "palinendophonia," associated with pure verbal palinacousis induced by a right inferior temporal lesion. Eur Neurol 2015;74: 219–221.

22 Fukutake T, Hattori T: Auditory illusions caused by a small lesion in the right medial geniculate body. Neurology 1998;51:1469–1471.

23 Masson C, Sztern A, Cambier J, Masson M: Palinacousis related to right temporoparietal hemorrhage. Presse Med 1993;22:596.

24 Robinson ME, Bialosky JE, Bishop MD, Price DD, George SZ: Supra-threshold scaling, temporal summation, and after-sensation: relationships to each other and anxiety/fear. J Pain Res 2010;3:25–32.
25 Bar-Shalita T, Vatine JJ, Yarnitsky D, Parush S, Weissman-Fogel I: Atypical central pain processing in sensory modulation disorder: absence of temporal summation and higher after-sensation. Exp Brain Res 2014;232:587–595.
26 Weeks SR, Anderson-Barnes VC, Tsao JW: Phantom limb pain: theories and therapies. Neurologist 2010; 16:277–286.
27 Brugger P: Supernumerary phantoms: a comment on Grossi, et al.'s (2002) spare thoughts on spare limbs. Percept Mot Skills 2003;97:3–10.
28 Itard JM: Mémoire sur quelques fonctions involontaires des appareils de la locomotion, de la préhension et de la voix. Arch Général Méd 1825;8:403–404.
29 De La Tourette G: Étude sur une affection nerveuse caractérisée par de l'incoordination motrice accompagnée d'écholalie et de coprolalie. Observation III. Arch Neurol 1885;9:19–42.
30 Souques AA: Palilalie. Rev Neurol 1908;16:340–342.
31 Brissaud E: Leçons sur les maladies nerveuses, 2ème serie. Paris, Ed Masson, 1899, vol 32, p 310.
32 Duffy JR: Motor Speech Disorders: Substrates, Differential Diagnosis, and Management. St. Louis, MO/London, Mosby, 1995.
33 Dietl T, Auer DP, Modell S, Lechner C, Trenkwalder C: Involuntary vocalisations and a complex hyperkinetic movement disorder following left side thalamic haemorrhage. Behav Neurol 2003;14:99–102.
34 Christman SS, Boutsen FR, Buckingham HW: Perseveration and other repetitive verbal behaviors: functional dissociations. Semin Speech Lang 2004;25: 295–307.
35 Max L, Guenther FH, Gracco VL, Ghosh SS, Wallace ME: Unstable or insufficiently activated internal models and feedback-biased motor control as sources of dysfluency: a theoretical model of stuttering. Contemp Issues Commun Sci Disord 2004;31:105–122.
36 Craig-McQuaide A, Akram H, Zrinzo L, Tripoliti E: A review of brain circuitries involved in stuttering. Front Hum Neurosci 2014;8:884.
37 Ghika J, Bogousslavsky J, Ghika-Schmid F, Regli F: "Echoing approval:" a new speech disorder. J Neurol 1996;243:633–637.
38 Dubois B, Slachevsky A, Pillon B, Beato R, Villalponda JM, Litvan I: "Applause sign" helps to discriminate PSP from FTD and PD. Neurology 2005;64: 2132–2133.
39 Cho YJ, Han SD, Song SK, Lee BI, Heo K: Palilalia, echolalia, and echopraxia-palipraxia as ictal manifestations in a patient with left frontal lobe epilepsy. Epilepsia 2009;50:1616–1619.
40 Lhermitte F: "Utilization behavior" and its relation to lesions of the frontal lobes. Brain 1983;106:237–255.
41 Lhermitte F, Pillon B, Serdaru M: Human autonomy and the frontal lobes. Part I: Imitation and utilization behaviour: a neuropsychological study of 75 patients. Ann Neurol 1986;19:326–334.
42 Ganos C, Ogrzal T, Schnitzler A, Münchau A: The pathophysiology of echopraxia/echolalia: relevance to Gilles de la Tourette syndrome. Mov Disord 2012; 27:1222–1229.
43 Ridley RM: The psychology of perserverative and stereotyped behaviour. Prog Neurobiol 1994;44: 221–231.
44 Ghika-Schmid F, Bogousslavsky J: The acute behavioral syndrome of anterior thalamic infarction: a prospective study of 12 cases. Ann Neurol 2000;48: 220–227.
45 Cooney RE, Joormann J, Eugène F, Dennis EL, Gotlib IH: Neural correlates of rumination in depression. Cogn Affect Behav Neurosci 2010;10:470–478.
46 Ferdek MA, van Rijn CM, Wyczesany M: Depressive rumination and the emotional control circuit: an EEG localization and effective connectivity study. Cogn Affect Behav Neurosci 2016;16:1099–1113.
47 Sierra M, Berrios GE: Flashbulb memories and other repetitive images: a psychiatric perspective. Compr Psychiatry 1999;40:115–125.
48 Politis M, Loane C: Reduplicative paramnesia: a review. Psychopathology 2012;45:337–343.
49 Langdon R, Connaughton E, Coltheart M: The Fregoli delusion: a disorder of person identification and tracking. Top Cogn Sci 2014;6:615–631.
50 Devinsky O: Delusional misidentifications and duplications: right brain lesions, left brain delusions. Neurology 2009;72:80–87.
51 Hurley S, Chater N: Perspective on Imitation: From Neuroscience to Social Science. Cambridge, MIT Press, 2005.
52 Iacoboni M: Mirroring People. New York, Farrar, Straus & Giroux, 2008.
53 Baxter MG: Involvement of medial temporal lobe structures in memory and perception. Neuron 2009; 61:667–677.
54 Suzuki WA: Perception and the medial temporal lobe: evaluating the current evidence. Neuron 2009; 61:657–666.
55 Baddeley AD, Allen RJ, Hitch GJ: Binding in visual working memory: the role of the episodic buffer. Neuropsychologia 2011;49:1393–1400.
56 Pulvermüller F, Garagnani M, Wennekers T: Thinking in circuits: toward neurobiological explanation in cognitive neuroscience. Biol Cybern 2014;108: 573–593.

57 Henderson A, Kim H, Kintz S, Frisco N, Wright HH: Working memory in aphasia: considering discourse processing and treatment implications. Semin Speech Lang 2017;38:40–51.
58 Bartolo A, Cubelli R, Della Sala S, Drei S: Pantomimes are special gestures which rely on working memory. Brain Cogn 2003;53:483–494.
59 Gabriel D, Wong TC, Nicolier M, Giustiniani J, Mignot C, Noiret N, Monnin J, Magnin E, Pazart L, Moulin T, Haffen E, Vandel P: Don't forget the lyrics! Spatiotemporal dynamics of neural mechanisms spontaneously evoked by gaps of silence in familiar and newly learned songs. Neurobiol Learn Mem 2016;132:18–28.
60 Yun SH, Lavin PJ, Schatz MP, Lesser RL: Topiramate-induced palinopsia: a case series and review of the literature. J Neuro Ophthalmol 2015;35:148–151.

Dr. Eloi Magnin
CMRR, Department of Neurology, Besançon University Hospital
Boulevard Fleming
FR–25000 Besançon (France)
E-Mail eloi.magnin@laposte.net

Bogousslavsky J (ed): Neurologic-Psychiatric Syndromes in Focus. Part I – From Neurology to Psychiatry.
Front Neurol Neurosci. Basel, Karger, 2018, vol 41, pp 40–49 (DOI: 10.1159/000475691)

Pathological Yawning, Laughing and Crying

Olivier Walusinski

Family Physician, Private Practice, Brou, France

Abstract

Yawning, laughing, and crying are normal physiological behaviors of humans in good health. As with all physiological behaviors, their deregulation can reveal disorders. Pathological yawning occurs in salvos of 10–20 successive yawns, and the number of yawns per day can exceed one hundred. After listing the functional etiologies, we will give the clinical keys for differentiating the most serious causes: iatrogenic, tumors, strokes, amyotrophic lateral sclerosis, and intracranial hypertension. Sudden, uncontrollable episodes of emotional display involving pathological laughing and crying (PLC) may be encountered in various neurological diseases: amyotrophic lateral sclerosis, multiple system atrophy (cerebellar), cerebrovascular disease, traumatic brain injuries, mass lesions in the cerebellopontine junction, and epilepsy. After describing the pathophysiology of PLC and the use of diagnostic scales for PLC, we will discuss the current treatments.

Introduction

Yawning, laughing, and crying are normal physiological behaviors of humans in good health. After a brief review of their physiology, we will show how and why these behaviors become pathological.

Yawning

Yawning is a stereotyped and often repetitive motor act characterized by gaping of the mouth, accompanied by a long inspiration of breath, a brief acme, and then a short expiration. Behavioral and neurophysiological studies provide converging evidence that yawning is linked to a low level of vigilance, before and after sleep episodes, when subjects are bored or engaged in repetitive and monotonous activities. Hunger or satiety also triggers yawning. Ethologists agree that all vertebrates yawn, in water, air, and land environments [1]. Yawning begins in fetuses as early as 12 weeks gestational age. Yawning frequency not only has a distinctive circadian distribution but also changes over the life span, being more frequent in infancy and decreasing with maturity [2]. Phylogenetically ancient and ontogenetically primitive, this motor behavior has been remarkably well preserved during evolution. It is closer to an emotional stereotypy than a reflex. Nevertheless, the purpose of this behavior remains controversial; relative to the abundance of hypotheses, there is little experimental data.

Yawning involves the paraventricular nucleus of the hypothalamus where a group of oxytocinergic neurons project to the hippocampus, the brainstem (reticular activating system or RAS and motor nuclei of cranial nerves V, VII, IX, X, XI, and XII), and the cervical spinal cord (phrenic nerves C1–C4). Numerous neurotransmitters and neurohormones are involved in the mediation of yawning, including oxytocin, acetylcholine, dopamine, glutamate, serotonin, GABA, adrenergics, ACTH, and αMSH [3]. Yawning appears to stimulate the structures responsible for cortical activation, and thus alertness, through the powerful musculoskeletal contraction of masticatory and cervical muscles [4].

History

Yawning has defied the human mind for centuries. Hippocrates, Évrart de Conty (1330–1405), Santorio Santorio (1561–1636), Danieli Sennerti (1572–1637), Herman Boerhaave (1668–1738), and Johannes de Gorter (1689–1762), for example, each advanced a theory in his time. From the release of tainted humor to the awakening of animal spirits and improved brain oxygenation, the metaphors that developed from these theories were all characterized by their popular success, which endured until the time of Jean-Martin Charcot (1825–1893) and continue their influence today. However, the neuromuscular theory, developed in the early 19th century and based on the experimental physiology of John M. Good (1764–1827), Pierre-Marie Flourens (1794–1867), Jean-Louis Brachet (1789–1858), and which Valentin Dumpert (working in Germany after World War I) explained in detail, remains the most relevant. Experimental pharmacology in the 20th century brought the neuromediators and subcortical structures involved in yawning and pandiculation to light [5].

Pathological Yawning

The analysis of clinical observations based on a century's worth of knowledge makes it possible to affirm the existence of pathological yawning [6]. The most frequent complaint is incomplete yawning leading to the frustration of a hedonic perception. Relaxation and anti-stress techniques help patients regain the proprioceptive rehabilitation of the body scheme that yawning generally gives. The absence of yawning remains exceptional, observed with certain extrapyramidal syndromes, opioid treatments or coffee overconsumption. Treating motor block episodes in Parkinson's

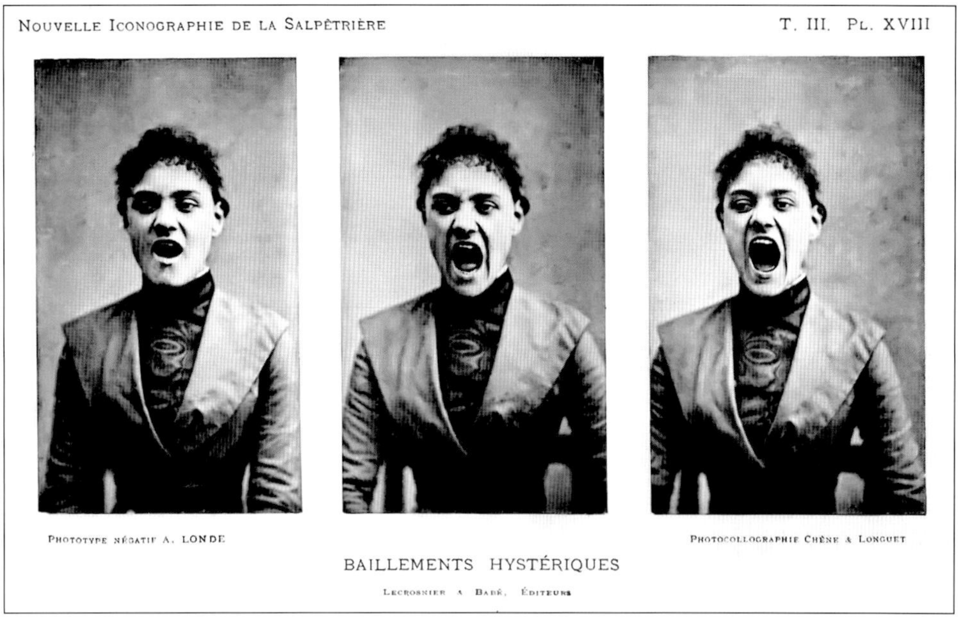

Fig. 1. Three photos in a series showing a hysterical woman yawning (she yawns 7 times per minute). By Albert Londe. In Gilles de la Tourette G, Huet E, Guinon G. Contribution à l'étude des bâillements hystériques. Nouvelle Iconographie de La Salpêtrière 1890; T.3:Pl. XVIII. Private collection of the author.

patients with apomorphine hydrochloride, a dopaminergic stimulant, triggers yawning as the first sign of unblocking.

A healthy person yawns three to ten times a day. Yawning becomes pathological when the frequency interferes with personal and social lives, often involving repetitive clusters of more than thirty yawns throughout the day. Excessive yawning may have functional or organic causes (Fig. 1).

Functional pathological yawning

The most common cause of frequent yawning is sleep debt, particularly in children and young adults. Drowsiness can be assessed using an Epworth score, to uncover a syndrome of sleep apnea. In children, where there is no sleep apnea caused by obstructive hypertrophy of the tonsils and adenoids, the diagnosis of attention deficit – hyperactivity disorder needs to be assessed.

Dyspepsia, or the sensation of a full stomach due to delayed emptying, and irritable bowel syndrome are "gut brain" disorders and should be considered in light of vasovagal disturbance and motion sickness. These disorders attest the hyperstimulation of the parasympathetic system and involve pallor, nausea, and salvos of yawning. Likewise, during invasive explorations, physicians need to watch for repetitive yawns to anticipate loss of consciousness. The feeling of hunger in non-diabetics or hypoglycemia in diabetics is accompanied by profuse sweating and repeated yawning.

Organic pathological yawning

Never associated with somnolence, increased yawning frequency due to serotoninergic antidepressant treatment is the type of pathological yawning most often observed in clinical practice. This symptom is often wrongly interpreted both by patients and physicians, who attribute it to asthenia and the persistence of a depressive state. Dosage is increased, whereas stopping the treatment would allow the symptom to disappear. Unfortunately, as this iatrogenic effect is rarely reported to drug safety agencies, there are no statistics to assess its frequency.

Detoxification after prolonged use in heavy coffee drinkers or opiate users is accompanied by a withdrawal syndrome that includes the occurrence of repetitive yawning over several days.

A large number of migraine sufferers experience repeated yawning as an aura before an attack. More rarely, the attack may end with drowsiness accompanied by yawning. The functional changes in hypothalamo-brainstem connectivity that partially explain migraine indicate involvement of the dopaminergic system, both in nociceptive pathways and in yawning, as well as during neuronal firing in the trigeminocervical complex [7].

Intracranial hypertension, whether related to stroke, tumor or head trauma, can be manifested by headaches and disturbed vigilance associated with salvos of yawns and convulsions, indicating herniation. Certain coma scores used in the US take into account the presence of yawning in these situations.

Yawning during stroke may be due to intracranial hypertension, but may also indicate damage to cortical and subcortical circuitry. In these cases, yawning acts as a mechanism of secondary vigilance stimulation controlled by the reticular formation of the brainstem. This mechanism also appears to be implicated in the yawning that occurs during partial seizure in temporal lobe epilepsy. The term "parakinesia brachialis oscitans" was coined to describe involuntary yawning-associated movements in a paralyzed arm during hemiplegia. After a stroke interrupts cortical control, the subjacent neurological structures revert to their ancestral functions, normally inhibited by the overlying cerebral structures as a result of evolution. During the diaphragm movement caused by yawning, the paralyzed arm receives motor stimulation from the lateral reticular nucleus of the medulla, which couples ventilation and locomotion in animals; the signal is not inhibited by the structure destroyed by ischemia. In the same way, despite paralysis of voluntary facial movements, yawning occurs during bilateral anterior opercular and locked-in syndromes. During acute anterior circulation stroke, yawning is associated with lesions of the insula and the caudate nucleus. Pathological yawning has also been associated with infratentorial lesions such as paramedian pontine infarcts. Finally, excessive yawning has been reported in amyotrophic lateral sclerosis and multiple sclerosis (MS) [8, 9].

Pathological Laughter and Crying

"Ce n'est pas toujours de tristesse qu'on pleure;
il entre bien des sortes de sentiments dans la composition des larmes"
"It is not always with sadness that we cry;
there are many sorts of feelings that enter into the composition of tears"
Madame de Sévigné, correspondence, 11 September 1680.

The larger part of our daily lives involves affective exhibition or generating various forms of body language, with no thought given to how or why. Laughter and crying are universal human vocalizations that evolved to shape the behavior of other people, similar to tears.

Scope of These Inappropriate Behaviors

Pathological laughing and crying (PLC) are episodes of uncontrollable outbursts of laughing and/or crying that either do not have an apparent motivating stimulus or are triggered by a stimulus that would not have led the subject to laugh or cry prior to the onset of the condition, without neglecting that the stimulus may have an emotional valence contrary to the emotional expression. Thus, PLC is a disorder of emotional expression, resulting in involuntary or disproportionate expression, rather than a primary disturbance of feelings. As a deficit in regulation and coordination of emotional expression, PLC differs from mood disorders, which are characterized by a pervasive and sustained problem of emotional experience. It remains unknown why other forms of affective display are not affected. While some patients exhibit problems with only laughter, others have problems with only crying, and still others exhibit problems with both. Although these patients do not laugh or cry at all times, when they do, the actual behavior of laughing or crying is often indistinguishable from normal acts of laughing and crying. The condition can occur continuously over several hours, with pauses only to draw breath. Then laughter, for example, may gradually give way to frequent giggles, low laughs, grimaces, and smiles, so that patients seem to be continuously muttering and laughing to themselves. Aware of their condition, patients are desperately embarrassed by their inappropriate emotional display, which they cannot voluntarily prevent or stop once it starts [10, 11].

Terminology

PLC is also known by other names: "pseudobulbar syndrome," "emotional lability," "emotional incontinence," and "involuntary emotional expression disorder."

History

In his 1812 thesis, Denis-Prudent Roy (1788– ?) listed various types of pathological laughter. In 1886, Oppenheim and Siemerling described cases of exaggerated emotional behavior in patients with lesions along the descending pathways to the brainstem ("Zwangslachen und Zwangsweinen") [12, 13]. According to Vladimir Mikhailovich

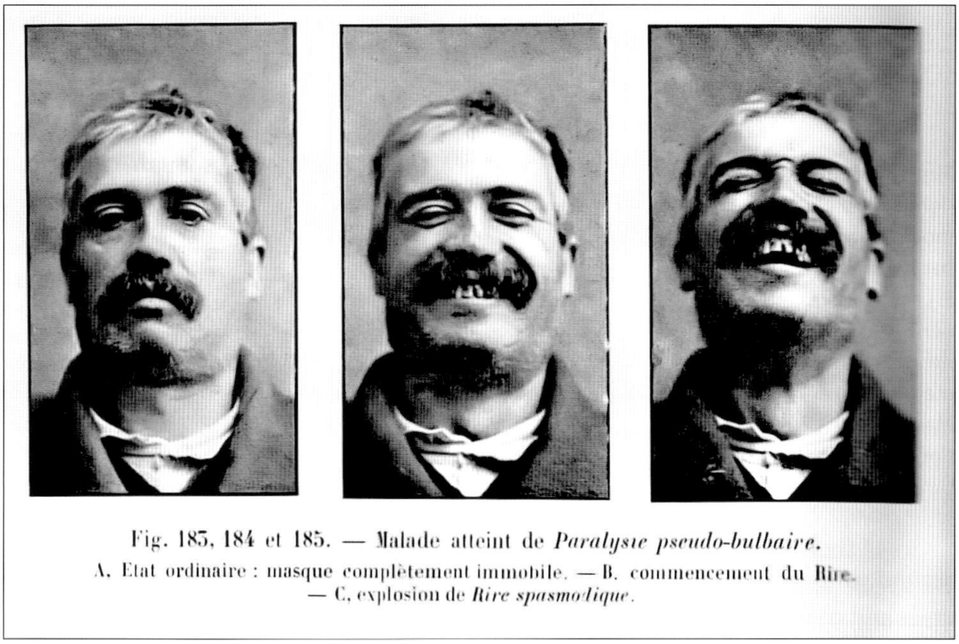

Fig. 2. A man affected with hemiplegia and spasmodic laughter ("pseudobulbar syndrome"). In Brisssaud E. Leçons sur les maladies nerveuses [XXI lesson: "Sur le rire et le pleurer spasmodique," p 460]. Paris, G. Masson, 1895. Private collection of the author.

Bekhterev (1857–1927) [14], PLC was caused by lesions in the anterior part of the thalamus, while Édouard Brissaud and his student Maurice Toulzac (1875– ?) suggested that the integrity of the thalamus was essential to the appearance of "spasmodic laughter or weeping" and that the causative lesion had to involve the anterior limb of the internal capsule, *"le faisceau psychique"* [15, 16] (Figs. 2, 3). The term "emotional incontinence," applied by psychiatrists at the time, may be accurate but is somewhat pejorative. In 1903, Charles Féré (1852–1907) coined the term *"fou rire prodromique"* (prodromal laughing fit) to describe explosive and continuous laughter that lacked a congruent emotional component and signaled an ischemic neurological deficit or chorea [17, 18]. Based on the cases reports of Bekhterev and Brissaud, Féré postulated that the centers for emotional expression were released from cortical inhibition. One explanation currently proposed is paradoxical embolism with a patent foramen ovale [19, 20]. Contemporary knowledge of pathological laughter dates from a 1956 article by Redvers Ironside (1899–1968) that compiled relevant scientific facts and studies [21].

Cerebral Localizations and Pathophysiology

The expression of laughter seems to depend on two partially independent neuronal pathways. The first pathway – the involuntary system – involves amygdaloid, thalamic and subthalamic areas, and the dorsal tegmental brainstem (triangle of Guillain-Mollaret which includes a component responsible for the short bursts in laughter). The

Bogousslavsky J (ed): Neurologic-Psychiatric Syndromes in Focus. Part I – From Neurology to Psychiatry.
Front Neurol Neurosci. Basel, Karger, 2018, vol 41, pp 50–60 (DOI: 10.1159/000475695)

Catastrophe Reaction and Emotionalism

Antonio Carota[a] · Julien Bogousslavsky[b]

[a]Clinique de Genolier, Genolier, and [b]Neurocenter, Swiss Medical Network, Clinique Valmont, Glion/Montreux, Switzerland

Abstract

The catastrophic reaction (CR; a disruptive and uncontrolled behavior triggered by anger, irritability, and hostility) and emotionalism (a condition of uncontrolled crying or laughing) are disorders of the emotional regulation and expression, the prevalence of which is underestimated in neurology. Their occurrence is an additional factor of poor outcome for neurologic patients. Although they have been recognized and completely described in their clinical manifestations more than a century ago, many issues remain unsolved regarding their pathogenesis and the respective role of the brain damage and psychological factors. Thus, if pathological crying and laughing can be linked to one or more lesions within the corticospinal tracts, the emotional lability and CR have uncertain connections within specific functional brain systems and seem to be influenced by personality factors or depression and anxiety generated by coping with a serious neurological disease. These epistemological difficulties are also the consequence of some methodological limits of the questionnaires and scales, which diagnose these disorders and for which the cut-off values between the normal and pathological condition could be questioned. Thus, their assessment requires new psychophysical. The CR and emotionalism manifest in association with several different neurological disease (degenerative, vascular, inflammatory, epilepsy) and psychiatric conditions as psychosis, mania, and mood disorders. Across these different diseases, the findings of common patterns of lesion location, cognitive dysfunction, emotional changes, and behavioral responses to new paradigms might clarify the pathogenesis and orient the treatment.

Introduction

Patients with different neurological diseases, and more specifically patients with stroke and aphasia, often manifest aggressiveness. The German neurologist, neuropsychologist, and psychiatrist Kurt Goldstein (1878–1965) first coined the term "catastrophic reaction" (CR), referring to a state of extreme confusion and anxiety involving the whole behavior (from here the sense of "catastrophic"), which is caused by the patient's sudden inability to perform certain tasks (i.e., a patient with aphasia facing a linguistic test). Thus, clinically, CR is an outburst of frustration, depression, and anger suddenly building up to an overwhelming degree with disruptive behaviors (shouting, cursing, hitting, kicking, and biting).

Within psychiatric taxonomies, this behavior is reminiscent of the intermittent explosive disorder (or episodic dyscontrol syndrome) in healthy adolescents, with the particularity that, in neurologic patients, rage and hostility of CR manifest as a reaction to the clinical evaluation.

In the 1960s, Tertian (1964) and Rossi and Rosadini (1967) reported that CR appears after barbiturates injection in the left carotid artery. In the 1970s, Gainotti confirmed in clinical studies the association among stroke, CR, and aphasia [1]. However, he suggested that the CR could be an appropriate emotional reaction to a particularly severe neurologic deficit and that it could interfere with the verbal assessment of post-stroke depression. In the 1990s, Starkstein et al. [2] attempted to validate a specific scale to inquire the presence and severity of the CR occurring in stroke patients and its link with mood disorders. However, the exact correlation among CR, aphasia, post-stroke depression, and emotionalism remains still to be defined in terms of neuronal circuits.

As well as CR, emotionalism too is a condition of emotional dysregulation. If CR corresponds to an uncontrolled and disruptive behavior triggered by anger, emotionalism is an uncontrolled behavior of crying and laughing triggered from either specific or unspecific stimuli. Thus, emotionalism indicates a condition of an increased frequency of crying (shedding tears, sobbing) or laughing in comparison to the patient's condition before the neurologic disorder. The onset of such crying or laughing occurs with little or no warning, the patient feels that the emotional expression goes beyond the normal control, and he or she might cry or laugh in social contexts when he or she would not have been previously behaving as such [3].

The first clinical description of emotionalism, such as laughing and crying out of control, dates to Darwin in 1872. An illustrative example of emotionalism in a neurologic patient can be traced historically to Cosimo I de' Medici (1519–1574) in the Renaissance [4]. Oppenheim first used the term pseudobulbar affect in 1911 [5].

In 1924, Wilson [6] formulated a general theory on the neural correlates of emotionalism in neurological disorders. This theory postulates the existence of 2 cortical systems connected by the corticospinal tracts to a hypothetical "crying-laughing" facial-respiratory center in the brainstem, responsible for the motor commands of crying and laughter. The first system, located in the frontal lobes and in the motor cortex, exercises a voluntary control, whereas the second, presumably connected to the limbic system, processes the emotional valence of the external stimuli and allows laughing and crying to emerge involuntarily. According to this theory, the insurgence of abnormal laughter and crying is due to the imbalance between the 2 systems and, for this reason, may manifest even after unilateral lesions.

consumption or with drug use. However, since several years, a growing group of authors also consider non-drug-related behaviors as being addictive in nature [1]. In general, addictive behavior may include different components, that is: (1) continued engagement in a given behavior despite its negative consequences; (2) compulsive engagement in this behavior; (3) reduced self-control over the engagement in this behavior; and (4) an appetitive urge or craving state prior to the engagement in this behavior. In the Diagnostic and Statistical Manual of Mental Disorders, version 5, many disorders conceptualized as "behavioral addictions" are currently categorized as "Impulse control disorders, not elsewhere classified" [2]. The understanding of the neuroanatomical networks underlying obsessive-compulsive disorders (OCD) has considerably increased (for reviews, see [3, 4]). Biological models of OCD propose anomalies in the serotonin pathways and dysfunctional circuits in the orbito-striatal area, including the caudate nucleus and the dorsolateral prefrontal cortex. Furthermore, structural imaging has evidenced abnormalities in cortico-striatal-thalamic-cortical circuits, such as decreased volume or increased grey matter density. Typical obsessional concerns such as contamination may result in compulsive washing or bathing; religious concerns result in compulsive praying and religious actions. Concerns for precision or symmetry result in compulsive ordering and arranging. Other obsessional concerns are harm to self or other people and result in compulsive checking and asking for reassurance. Finally, hoarding may be the result of obsessional saving concerns.

A meta-analysis of brain imaging results in adults has suggested that OCD symptoms may rely on dysfunctional activity within the orbitofrontal cortex and the caudate nucleus [5]. However, other regions of the brain might also play a role in OCD, in particular the temporal lobe [6, 7] and the amygdala [8].

Disease Pathogenesis

OCD Symptoms after Brain Injury

Addictive and obsessive-compulsive behavior following acquired brain lesions has been rarely reported. Several single case reports, or small case series, described OCD following different types of brain injury, such as traumatic brain injury, cerebrovascular accidents, brain tumors, or infections of the brain (for review, see [9, 10]). OCD as a psychiatric disease has a lifetime prevalence of approximately 2.5–3% [11, 12] in the general population.

Silver et al. [13] found, in a large sample of the general population, an association between a history of brain injury and the lifetime risk of developing a psychiatric illness, including OCD. In this study, the lifetime prevalence for OCD was 4.7% in patients with brain injury, compared to 2.3% in patients without head injury. However, the causal nature of this association, and the temporal relationship between the injury and the development of the symptomatology, remains unclear. Berthier et al.

[14, 15] described a case series of 10 patients with OCD following traumatic brain injury. The researchers concluded that a specific pattern of behavior and cognitive impairment was common to all the patients of this group, including aggressive behavior, contamination, and sexual obsessions. Furthermore, the patients showed obsessive cleaning, checking, and repeating compulsions. Unusual features, such as obsessional slowness and compulsive exercising, were also found. These symptoms were accompanied by cognitive impairment on measures of general intellectual ability, memory, and executive control function [15]. These cognitive impairments, while thought to be specific to OCD following traumatic brain injury, may be similar to those observed in patients with traumatic brain injury per se, in the absence of OCD. Lesion localization in OCD following traumatic brain injury includes the orbitofrontal, the anterior cingulate, and the anterior temporal (left and right) cortex [15–18]. Furthermore, the caudate nucleus and the globus pallidus may also be involved.

OCD following stroke is rare, and only few case studies have been published. In their case series, Berthier et al. [14] described the case of a patient who suffered from a small ischemic infarction within the right posterior putamen. Other cases of OCD following unilateral, left-sided ischemic infarctions or hemorrhages in the area of the basal ganglia [19–21], or bilateral infarctions of the globus pallidus and of the caudate nucleus [22, 23], have also been described.

The case described by Simpson and Baldwin [24] is particularly interesting, since this patient suffered from a right hemispheric inferior parietal infarction, but single-photon emission CT also showed an additional decrease in cerebral blood flow with in the right hemispheric basal ganglia area. This case thus illustrates the potentially important role of functional disconnections in the development of OCD symptoms after acquired brain lesions, that is, the dysfunctional changes in cerebral regions distant from the anatomical lesion site. OCD symptoms have also been reported after infarcts within the territory of the left middle cerebral artery [25, 26] and after right posterior frontal infarctions [27].

Hyperphagia

Isolated hyperphagia, that is, the abnormally increased appetite for consumption of food, has seldom been reported following head injury. Hyperphagia is mostly described following lesions of the hypothalamic-pituitary system, such as following lesions of the ventromedial hypothalamic and paraventricular nuclei [28–30]. Transient hyperphagia was also described after a left medial thalamic infarction [31], suggesting a transient thalamocortical dysfunction due to an impairment of the connections between the medial thalamus and the frontal or temporal lobes.

Furthermore, eating disorders may also occur due to tumors within the temporal cortex, in temporal lobe epilepsy, in advanced states of dementia with neuronal loss within the medial temporal lobes, or in anti-NMDA receptor encephalitis [32–34]. Hyperphagia is also part of the Klüver-Bucy syndrome [35].

Gourmand Syndrome
The gourmand syndrome (GS) was originally described by Regard and Landis [36]. Patients with GS show a new, intense preoccupation with food, and a preference for fine eating. The authors described the cases of 36 patients with GS, out of which 34 patients (94%) had a lesion in the right hemisphere. Most of these patients had a frontal or temporal lesion. Thirty of the 36 patients with GS had a temporal damage (83%), and twelve patients had an additional parietal damage (33%). The etiology of the brain lesions was a tumor in 14 patients (39%), a vascular lesion in 12 patients (33%), epilepsy in 8 patients (22%), and traumatic brain injury in 2 patients (5%). Gallo et al. [37] described the case of a patient who presented with GS and had a lesion of the right amygdala and of the right temporal pole. Finally, Kurian et al. [38] reported a case of GS in a 10-year-old boy with epilepsy following a right temporoparietal hemorrhagic lesion. In conclusion, GS can be considered as a form of benign hyperphagia syndrome, occurring mainly after right temporal lesions. The etiology of GS is often tumoral or epileptic. This led to the speculation that the neuronal activity beyond the lesion triggers the activation of a wider network, which finally results in the development of a complex eating behavior and in the peculiar attitudes toward eating [38].

Klüver-Bucy Syndrome
The Klüver-Bucy syndrome (KBS) is a constellation of cognitive dysfunctions including indiscriminate dietary behavior and hyperphagia, hyperorality, hypermetamorphosis (i.e., the tendency to react to every visual stimulus), the inability to recognize the emotional significance of objects, altered emotional behavior (particularly placidity), hypersexuality, and amnesia (anterograde, retrograde, or global) [35].

A full-blown form of KBS rarely occurs in humans [39]. Partial KBS forms are diagnosed when 3 of the aforementioned symptoms are present. KBS in humans is rather uncommon, with fewer than 200 publications in PubMed reporting its occurrence [40].

KBS was reported after a variety of different pathologies, such as trauma, tumor, herpes encephalitis, hypoxia, multiple sclerosis, lupus erythematosus, but also in neurodegenerative diseases such as Alzheimer's disease and frontotemporal dementia (for a review, see [40]).

Originally, it was believed that KSB is provoked by a bilateral damage of the anterior part of the temporal lobes, especially of the amygdala. However, KSB can also occur after unilateral left temporal lesions [41], or unilateral right temporal lesions [42]. Interestingly, this patient presented with hyperphagia, placidity, and hyposexuality. Furthermore, KBS was also reported in a patient with isolated bilateral hippocampal atrophy following a status epilepticus [43]. Lesions involving the neuronal connections originating from the amygdala may also provoke KBS [44]. Finally, lesions of the right temporal lobe and of the right orbitofrontal regions, including the bilateral rectal and the medial orbital gyri, may also provoke KBS [45].

Kleptomania

Kleptomania is defined as the "recurrent failure to resist impulses to steal objects that are not needed for personal use or for their monetary value." The patients suffering from kleptomania feel an increasing sense of tension immediately before committing the theft. Several authors [46, 47] suggested that this syndrome is associated with strong obsessive and compulsive features, and may therefore be considered as part of the spectrum of OCD. A review of the literature shows that several case reports of kleptomania associated with focal, organic brain injury have been reported. Kleptomania has been described in relation to frontal lobes dysfunction [48], right parietal tumors [49], subarachnoid hemorrhage with consecutive right basal forebrain lesions [50], contusion of left temporal lobe [51], and right fronto-limbic lesions [52]. The last mentioned case [52] is particularly interesting. Although electroencephalography did not show any epileptiform activity, the patient also exhibited behavioral symptoms of the Gastaut-Geschwind syndrome (GGS), commonly associated with temporal lobe epilepsy. For instance, he showed circumstantial behavior (i.e., the tendency to answer questions by providing excessive and unneeded details), and he presented a need to discuss his religious and moral beliefs, his dislikes, and his preferences. Furthermore, he showed hypergraphia, excessively writing about his preoccupation with religious ideas, justice, and altruism. We recently had the opportunity to observe a similar case, presenting with the unusual combination of kleptomania and hyper-religiosity, which we will describe in the following.

Original Case Report

We describe the case of a 56-year-old man, who suffered from a herpes simplex encephalitis, which resulted in a mainly right-sided lesion of the temporal lobe, including the anterior pole, and in a small left-sided temporal lesion (Fig. 1). The patient showed persistent neuropsychological deficits, mainly involving an impairment of the non-verbal memory, an executive dysfunction, reduced cognitive flexibility, and perseveration. Furthermore, the patient showed word finding impairments, particularly for words belonging to low-frequency object classes. The patient also presented with personality changes, such as self-neglect, diffuse and digressive communication, and reduced empathy. These personality changes led to a divorce. After the acute phase, the patient also started to repeatedly steal small amounts of money from the office of one of his friends.

Subsequently, the office of the patient's friend was monitored by the police, and then the patient was arrested for theft. He was not able to explain the reasons for his acts, and he could return the stolen money, since he did not spend it. At the same time, the patient felt the compulsion to visit churches (sometimes up to 10 churches a day), to pray, and to light votive candles. Before the encephalitis, the patient was not religious. The patient did not show any sign of hypergraphia, and electroencephalography did

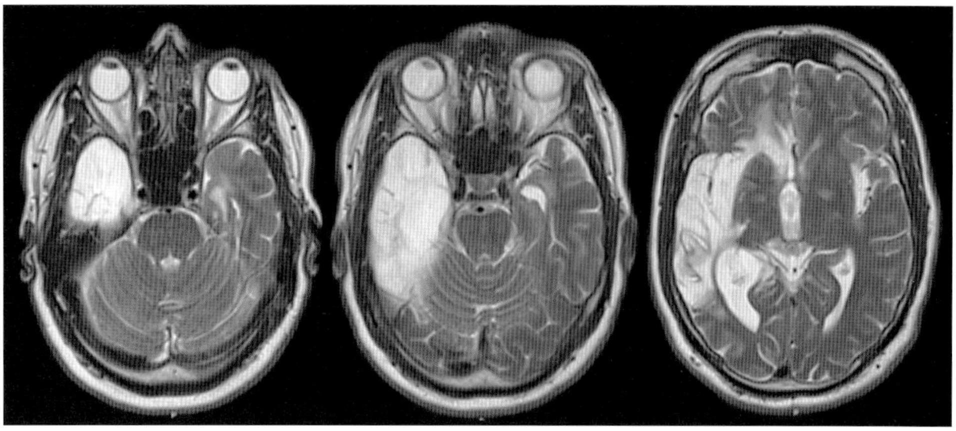

Fig. 1. Axial slices of T2 weighted MRI, showing defects in the right hemispheric temporal lobe and, to a lesser degree, also in the left hemispheric temporal pole and lobe, after herpes simplex encephalitis.

not show any epileptiform activity suggestive of a classical GGS. This single case thus shows an unusual combination of kleptomania and hyper-religiosity, which is similar to the one described by Nyffeler and Regard [52].

Gastaut-Geschwind Syndrome

The clinical picture of the GGS comprises hypergraphia, hyposexuality, hyper-religiosity, increased concern with philosophical matters, irritability, mood lability, and viscosity (i.e., the striking preoccupation with details and concerns over moral and ethical issues) [53]. Waxman and Geschwind [53] developed the concept of GSS as an organic brain syndrome, secondary to a temporal lobe/limbic dysfunction, and due to temporal lobe epilepsy.

A chronic stimulation of the amygdala, due to seizure activity, may lead to altered behavior and heightened emotionality during the interictal period. This behavior is what Geschwind described as an epileptic personality or as an interictal behavior. Bear and Fedio [54] speculated that the epileptic focus somehow led to enhanced associations between affect and stimuli, a so-called "functional hyper-connection" between neocortical and limbic structures. Waxman and Geschwind [53] counterposed this clinical picture both with the frontal lobe syndrome and with the KBS, having some characteristics almost opposite to the latter. The effects of removing brain tissue or chronically stimulating the same regions appear to result in the opposite symptomatology. Already Gastaut et al. [55] noted that these behavioral expressions were distinctly different from the effects of bilateral anterior temporal lesions as observed in the KBS. The GGS has been intensively debated in the literature, and the results of a study by Hoffmann [56] question the pathophysiology underlying this syndrome. In a group of 2,389 stroke patients, he found 5 patients with acute, isolated right temporal lobe stroke, who presented with GGS. Thus, GGS symptoms may also be provoked acutely after stroke. Isolated right temporal lobe strokes are relatively rare, and the temporal lobe is very often involved in larger vascular lesions within the middle cerebral artery territory, the most frequently involved artery in stroke. However, to the best of our knowledge, there are no reports concerning GGS after larger strokes involving simultaneously the temporal and frontal lobes. One may thus speculate that intra-hemispheric interactions (between temporal and frontal lobes) are important for the occurrence of the GGS.

Hypergraphia

Hypergraphia following focal brain lesion is a rare phenomenon, and seems to mainly occur after right hemispheric lesions. Yamadory et al. [57] described the cases of 5 stroke patients with hypergraphia, who produced linguistically correct, but semantically loose, writing. Writing behavior in these patients had several common features. The patients had lesions in the perisylvian cortico-subcortical or thalamic region of the right hemisphere. Imamura's patient [58] presented with hypergraphia and had a metastatic brain tumor localized in the right hemisphere. A case of hypergraphia following a cingulate lesion within the right anterior cerebral artery territory has been reported by Carota et al. [59].

As mentioned before, hypergraphia is also a part of the GGS. Hypergraphia may also have positive implications, as in the case of famous writers such as Dostoevsky, or in philosophers such as Kierkegaard, who had a conspicuous creative output. Hypergraphia due to stroke or due to temporal lobe epilepsy seems to present different distinctive features. Based on their case series, Okamura et al. [60] attempted to classify the characteristic features and differences between hypergraphia associated with stroke and temporal lobe epilepsy. Based on the dimensions "attitude" and "structure" of writing, they proposed that hypergraphia after stroke is poorly attentive, half involuntary, and loose in association. In contrast, hypergraphia in temporal lobe epilepsy is extremely attentive, compulsive-careful, and meticulously detailed. The structure of writing after stroke is irregular, concerning letter size and spatial arrangement, whereas in temporal lobe epilepsy regular letter size and spatial arrangement dominate. Finally, hypergraphia appears after stroke acutely or subacutely and is a transient phenomenon. In temporal lobe epilepsy, hypergraphia develops over years.

Hyper-Religiosity

Hyper-religiosity is a rare manifestation following a focal brain lesion. Most commonly, it occurs as a part of the GGS. The pathophysiology underlying hyper-religiosity is complex and not fully understood. Religiosity in the context of epilepsy is thought to be related to the limbic system, due to its association with the temporal lobe and its functional role in emotional regulation. Kindling might be one of the ways hyper-religiosity develops, as it is believed that the activation and strengthening of limbic-cortical connections may occur in patients with temporal epilepsy [61]. Wuerfel et al. [62] evaluated the hippocampal volumes in the MRI images of 33 patients with refractory epilepsy, and found that patients with hyper-religiosity showed a smaller right hippocampus. However, there was no correlation between hippocampal atrophy and other components of the GGS syndrome, suggesting that the right hippocampus may play a role in the development of religiosity per se [62]. Hyper-religiosity is also a behavioral symptom observed in neurodegenerative diseases. In patients with frontotemporal dementia, Chan et al. [63] found that the symptoms distinctive of a patient subgroup with right temporal lobe atrophy included hyper-religiosity, visual hallucinations, and cross-modal sensory experiences. Finally, Carmona-Bayonasa et al. [64] described the case of a patient with hyper-religiosity due to a malignant brain tumor localized in the right prefrontal cortex and the right temporal lobe.

Conclusions

In general, obsessive-compulsive and addictive behavior following focal brain lesions are rarely described in the literature. In some cases, the causal relationship between lesions and symptoms is not unequivocal, and premorbid conditions may also play a role (e.g., [10, 13]). The overview provided in this chapter also shows that addictive or obsessive-compulsive symptoms in patients with focal lesions may occur in isolation, or in unusual combinations, challenging the 'classical' concepts of the Klüver-Bucy or of the GGS. For future studies, a more careful and systematic analysis of the different levels of neurological deficits is needed, from an elementary neurological level, to a more complex cognitive-neurological and neuropsychiatric level [56].

Acknowledgement

We would like to thank Prof. Klemens Gutbrod for examining the patient described in the case report.

Further Readings

van Vugt P, Paquier P, Kees L, Cras P: Increased writing activity in neurological conditions: a review and clinical study. J Neurol Neurosurg Psychiatr 1996;61:510–514.

References

1 Holden C: 'Behavioral' addictions: do they exist? Science 2001;294:980–982.

2 Grant JE, Potenza MN: Overview of the impulse control disorders not elsewhere classified and limitations of knowledge; in Grant JE, Potenza MN (eds): The Oxford Handbook of Impulse Control Disorders. New York, Oxford University Press, 2012, pp 3–10.

3 Stein DJ: Obsessive-compulsive disorder. Lancet 2002;360:397–405.

4 Abramowitz JS, Taylor S, McKay D: Obsessive-compulsive disorder. Lancet 2009;374:491–499.

5 Whiteside S, Port J, Abramowitz J: A meta-analysis of functional neuroimaging in obsessive-compulsive disorder. Psychiatry Res 2004;132:69–79.

6 Hugo F, van Heerden B, Zungu-Dirwayi N, Stein DJ: Functional brain imaging in obsessive-compulsive disorder secondary to neurological lesions. Depress Anxiety 1999;10:129–136.
7 Zungu-Dirwayi N, Hugo F, van Heerden BB, Stein DJ: Are musical obsessions a temporal lobe phenomenon? J Neuropsychiatry Clin Neurosci 1999;11: 398–400.
8 Szeszko PR, Robinson D, Alvir JM, Bilder RM, Lencz T, Ashtari M, Wu H, Bogerts B: Orbital frontal and amygdala volume reductions in obsessive-compulsive disorder. Arch Gen Psychiatry 1999;56:913–919.
9 Etcharry-Bouyx F, Dubas F: Obsessive-compulsive disorders in association with focal brain lesions; in Bogousslavsky J, Cummings J (eds): Behavior and Mood Disorders in Focal Brain Lesions. Cambridge, Cambridge University Press, 2000, pp 304–326.
10 Coetzer BR: Obsessive-compulsive disorder following brain injury: a review. Int J Psychiatry Med 2004; 34:363–377.
11 Jenike MA: An update on obsessive-compulsive disorder. Bull Menninger Clin 2001;65:4–25.
12 Karno M, Golding JM, Sorenson SB, Burnam MA: The epidemiology of obsessive-compulsive disorder in five US communities. Arch Gen Psychiatry 1988; 45:1094–1099.
13 Silver JM, Kramer R, Greenwald S, Weissman M: The association between head injuries and psychiatric disorders: findings from the new have NIMH epidemiologic catchment area study. Brain Inj 2001;15: 935–945.
14 Berthier ML, Kulisevsky J, Gironell A, Heras JA: Obsessive-compulsive disorder associated with brain lesions: clinical phenomenology, cognitive function, and anatomic correlates. Neurology 1996;47:353–361.
15 Berthier ML, Kulisevsky JJ, Gironell A, Lopez OL: Obsessivecompulsive disorder and traumatic brain injury: behavioral, cognitive, and neuroimaging findings. Neuropsychiatry Neuropsychol Behav Neurol 2001;14:23–31.
16 Ogai M, Iyo M, Mori N, Takei N: A right orbitofrontal region and OCD symptoms: a case report. Acta Psychiatr Scand 2005;111:74–77; discussion 76–77.
17 Bilgic B, Baral-Kulaksizoglu I, Hanagasi H, Saylan M, Aykutlu E, Gurvit H, Emre M: Obsessive-compulsive disorder secondary to bilateral frontal damage due to a closed head injury. Cog Behav Neurol 2004;17:118–120.
18 Hofer H, Frigerio S, Frischknecht E, Gassmann D, Gutbrod K, Müri RM: Diagnosis and treatment of an obsessive-compulsive disorder following traumatic brain injury: a single case and review of the literature. Neurocase 2013;19:390–400.
19 Carmin CN, Wiegartz PS, Yunus U, Gillock KL: Treatment of late-onset OCD following basal ganglia infarct. Depress Anxiety 2002;15:87–90.
20 Thobois S, Jouanneau E, Bouvard M, Sindou M: Obsessive-compulsive disorder after unilateral caudate nucleus bleeding. Acta Neurochir 2004;146:1027–1031; discussion 1031.
21 Weilburg JB, Mesulam MM, Weintraub S, Buonanno F, Jenike M, Stakes JW: Focal striatal abnormalities in a patient with obsessive-compulsive disorder. Arch Neurol 1989;46:233–235.
22 Rodrigo Escalona P, Adair JC, Roberts BB, Graeber DA: Obsessive-compulsive disorder following bilateral globuspallidusinfarction. Biol Psychiatry 1997;42:410–412.
23 Williams AC, Owen C, Heath DA: A compulsive movement disorder with cavitation of caudate nucleus. J Neurol Neurosurg Psychiatry 1988;51:447–448.
24 Simpson S, Baldwin B: Neuropsychiatry and SPECT of an acute obsessive-compulsive syndrome patient. Br J Psychiatry 1995;166:390–392.
25 Mahendran R: Obsessive compulsive disorder following left middle cerebral artery infarct. Singapore Med J 2000;41:498–499.
26 Borras L, Swine B, Constant EL, Huguelet P: Obsessive-compulsive disorder following left middle cerebral artery infarct. Acta Neuropsychiatrica 2007;19:71–72.
27 Swoboda KJ, Jenike MA: Frontal abnormalities in a patient with obsessive-compulsive disorder: the role of structural lesions in obsessive-compulsive behaviour. Neurology 1995;45:2130–2134.
28 Coffex RJ: Hypothalamic and basal forebrain germinoma presenting with amnesia and hyperphagia. Surg Neurol 1989;31:228–233.
29 Shinoda M, Tsugu A, Oda S, Masuko A, Yamaguchi T, Yamaguchi T, Tsuganc R, Sato O: Development of akinetic mutism and hyperphagia after left thalamic and right hypothalamic lesions. Childs Nerv Syst 1993;9:243–245.
30 Celesia GG, Archer CR, Chung HD: Hyperphagia and obesity. Relationship to medial hypothalamic lesions. JAMA 1981;246:151–153.
31 Cerrato P, Grasso M, Azzaro C, Baima C, Giraudo M, Rizzuto A, Lentini A, Perozzo P, Bergamasco B, Sorrentino G: Transient compulsive hyperphagia in a patient with a thalamic infarct. J Neurol Neurosurg Psychiatry 2004;75:1364–1365.
32 Keene J, Hope T: Natural history of hyperphagia and other eating changes in dementia. Int J Geriatr Psychiatry 1998;13:700–706.
33 Castano B, Capdevila E: Eating disorders in patients with traumatic brain injury: a report of four cases. NeuroRehabilitation 2010;27:113–116.
34 Perogamvros L, Schnider A, Leemann B: The role of NMDA receptors in human eating behavior: evidence from a case of anti-NMDA receptor encephalitis. Cogn Behav Neurol 2012;25:93–97.
35 Klüver H, Bucy PC: An analysis of certain effect of bilateral temporal lobectomy in the rhesus monkey, with special reference to "Psychic blindness." J Psychol 1938;5:33–54.

36 Regard M, Landis T: "Gourmand syndrome": eating passion associated with right anterior lesions. Neurology 1997;48:1185–1190.
37 Gallo M, Gámiz F, Perez-García M, Del Moral RG, Rolls ET: Taste and olfactory status in a gourmand with a right amygdala lesion. Neurocase 2014;20:421–433.
38 Kurian M, Schmitt-Mechelke T, Korff C, Delavelle J, Landis T, Seeck M: "Gourmand syndrome" in a child with pharmacoresistant epilepsy. Epilepsy Behav 2008;13:413–415.
39 Trimble MR, Mendez MF, Cummings JL: Neuropsychiatric symptoms from the temporolimbic lobes. J Neuropsychiatry Clin Neurosci 1997;9:429–438.
40 Caro MA, Jimenez XF: Mesiotemporal disconnection and hypoactivity in Klüver-Bucy syndrome: case series and literature review. J Clin Psychiatry 2016;77:e982–e988.
41 Ghika-Schmid F, Assal G, De Tribolet N, Regli F: Klüver-Bucy syndrome after left anterior temporal resection. Neuropsychologia 1995;33:101–113.
42 Bates GD, Sturman SG: Unilateral temporal lobe damage and the partial Kluver-Bucy syndrome. Behav Neurol 1995;8:103–107.
43 Park HK, Kim KJ, Moon HJ, Kim SJ, Yun CH, Park SH: Klüver-Bucy syndrome with isolated bilateral hippocampal atrophy following status epilepticus. J Epilepsy Res 2012;2:10–12.
44 Hayman LA, Rexer JL, Pavol MA, Strite D, Meyers CA: Klüver-Bucy syndrome after bilateral selective damage of amygdala and its cortical connections. J Neuropsychiatry Clin Neurosci 1998;10:354–358.
45 Yoneoka Y, Takeda N, Inoue A, Ibuchi Y, Kumagai T, Sugai T, Takeda KI, Ueda K: Human Kluver-Bucy syndrome following acute subdural haematoma. Acta Neurochir (Wien) 2004;146:1267–1270.
46 McElroy SL, Pope HG Jr, Hudson JI, Keck PE Jr, White KL: Kleptomania: a report of 20 cases. Am J Psychiatry 1991;148:652–657.
47 Hollander E, Wong CM: Obsessive-compulsive spectrum disorders. J Clin Psychiatry 1995;56(suppl 4):3–6; discussion 53–55.
48 Kozian R: [Kleptomania in frontal lobe lesion]. Psychiatr Prax 2001;28:98–99.
49 Chiswick D: Shoplifting, depression and an unusual intracranial lesion (a case report). Med Sci Law 1976;16:266–268.
50 Gossling HW, Rosin J: [Kleptomania before and after spontaneous subarachnoid hemorrhage – a neuropsychodynamic case report]. Fortschr Neurol Psychiatr 1994;62:164–168.

Prof. Dr. med. René M. Müri
Department of Neurology, University Neurorehabilitation
Freiburgstrasse 8
CH–3010 Bern (Switzerland)
E-Mail rene.mueri@insel.ch

51 Aizer A, Lowengrub K, Dannon PN: Kleptomania after head trauma: two case reports and combination treatment strategies. Clin Neuropharmacol 2004;27:211–215.
52 Nyffeler T, Regard M: Kleptomania in a patient with a right frontolimbic lesion. Neuropsychiatry Neuropsychol Behav Neurol 2001;14:73–76.
53 Waxman SG, Geschwind N: The interictal behavior syndrome of temporal lobe epilepsy. Arch Gen Psychiatry 1975;32:1580–1586.
54 Bear D, Fedio P: Quantitative analysis of interictal behaviour in temporal lobe epilepsy. Archives of Neurology 1977;34:454–467.
55 Gastaut H, Morin G, Leserve N: Etude du comportement des epileptiques psycho-moteurs dans l'intervalle de leurs crises. Ann Medico-Psychol 1955;113:1–27.
56 Hoffmann M: Isolated right temporal lobe stroke patients present with Geschwind Gastaut syndrome, frontal network syndrome and delusional misidentification syndromes. Behav Neurol 2008;20:83–89.
57 Yamadori A, Mori E, Tabuchi M, Kudo Y, Mitani Y: Hypergraphia: a right hemisphere syndrome. Neurol Neurosurg Psychiatry 1986;49:160–164.
58 Imamura T, Yamadori A, Tsuburaya: Hypergraphia associated with a brain tumour of the right cerebral hemisphere. Neurol Neurosurg Psychiatry 1992;55:25–27.
59 Carota A, Annoni JM, Combremont P, Clarke S, Bogousslavsky J: Hypergraphia, verbal aspontaneity and post-stroke depression secondary to right cingulate and corpus callosum infarction. J Neurol 2003;250:508–510.
60 Okamura T, Motomura N, Asaba H, Sakai T, Fukai M, Mori E, Yamadori A: Hypergraphia in temporal lobe epilepsy – compared with stroke of the right cerebral hemisphere. Jpn J Psychiatry Neurol 1989;43:524–525.
61 Dolgoff-Kaspar R, Ettinger AB, Golub SA, Perrine K, Harden C, Croll SD: Numinous-like auras and spirituality in persons with partial seizures. Epilepsia 2011;52:640–644.
62 Wuerfel J, Krishnamoorthy ES, Brown RJ, Lemieux L, Koepp M, Tebartz van Elst L, Trimble MR: Religiosity is associated with hippocampal but not amygdala volumes in patients with refractory epilepsy. J Neurol Neurosurg Psychiatry 2004;75:640–642.
63 Chan D, Anderson V, Pijnenburg Y, Whitwell J, Barnes J, Scahill R, Stevens JM, Barkhof F, Scheltens P, Rossor MN, Fox NC: The clinical profile of right temporal lobe atrophy. Brain 2009;132(pt 5):1287–1298.
64 Carmona-Bayonas A, Jiménez-Fonseca P, Vázquez Olmos C, Vega Villar J: Hyperreligiosity in malignant brain tumors: a case report and accompanying bibliographic review. Neurocase 2017;23:88–95.

Bogousslavsky J (ed): Neurologic-Psychiatric Syndromes in Focus. Part I – From Neurology to Psychiatry.
Front Neurol Neurosci. Basel, Karger, 2018, vol 41, pp 71–76 (DOI: 10.1159/000475693)

Hypersexuality in Neurological Disorders: From Disinhibition to Impulsivity

M. Béreau

Department of Neurology, CHRU Besançon, Besançon, France

Abstract

Little is known about the neurological control of human sexual behavior. Investigating and measuring this behavior by using quantitative and objective methods is difficult. Insights from lesion studies contribute to analyze the effects of neurological disorders on human sexual behavior. In this chapter, we focus on frontal lobe lesions, brain injuries, epilepsia, dementia, and Parkinson disease to describe human sexual behavior disorders, in order to highlight cortical and subcortical brain regions and neural networks involved in human sexual behavior.

Introduction

Human sexual behavior is complex and depends on many factors, including individual and societal values. There is currently no consensual definition of normal and pathological sexual behavior. However, case report and functional imaging studies have highlighted brain regions involved in the control of human sexual behavior. Such behaviors were initially considered as the result of general disinhibition revealing premorbid personality. Further studies in dementia and Parkinson disease have shown that these behaviors were also related to the reward system dysfunction.

Hypersexuality Following Brain Lesions

Studies of patients with brain lesions present an opportunity to identify brain regions implicated in human sexual behavior. In 1954, Jarvie et al. [1] described 6 cases of penetrating brain wound in which disinhibition appeared after the involvement of frontal lobes. In 3 cases, disinhibition occurs predominantly in sexual behavior. Sexual disinhibition included obscene language, sexual intercourses, masturbation, indecent exposure, and exhibitionistic practices. In most cases, patients were aware of their behavioral change. Interestingly, sexual behavior was not necessary associated with other features described in the frontal lobe syndrome, especially loss of initiative and intellectual impairment. Authors considered disinhibition as a disturbance of the mechanisms responsible for the control of socially appropriate behaviors. They hypothesized that breakdown in the control of these behaviors after frontal lobe injury was due to the destruction of an inhibitory process which revealed pre-morbid tendencies.

In 1986, Miller et al. [2] described 8 cases with hypersexuality or altered sexual preference following brain injury due to cerebrovascular disease, seizure or viral encephalitis. In these cases, patients had various sexual behavior disturbances characterized by either hypersexuality including public masturbation, increased sexual drive, verbal preoccupation with sex, neither altered sexual preferences marked by pedophilia, and change from hetero to homosexual preference. Disinhibition and hypersexuality followed medial basal frontal or diencephalic lesions of the brain whereas altered sexual preference followed limbic structure lesions. In these cases, sexual disinhibition was often associated with a general disinhibition of behavior.

Kleine Levin Syndrome

Kleine Levin syndrome (KLS) is a rare disease characterized by recurrent episodes of hypersomnia associated in various degrees with behavioral and cognitive disturbances, including hyperphagia and hypersexuality [3]. KLS occurs in an estimated 1–5 per million individuals worldwide. The disease affects predominantly teenagers and is rare over the age of 30 years. Boys are 4 times more likely than girls to be diagnosed with KLS. KLS was first described by Kleine (1925) [4] and Levine (1936) [5] who identified the recurring nature of episodes of hypersomnia and the association with "morbid hunger." Critchley and Hoffman further defined this syndrome as a distinct entity and gave the eponymous name to the disease [6]. They distinguished between KLS and narcolepsy, a more common sleep disorder. They also suggested that the pathophysiological process involved the hypothalamus.

Since then, many case reports have been published. Although the classic triad of hypersomnia, hyperphagia, and hypersexuality arose, it has been found that these symptoms were not always present [3]. In a large case series, less than half of KLS patients presented with all three symptoms [7]. Arnulf et al. [8] carried out a systematic review of 186 KLS cases in the literature. Sixty-five patients (43%) had symptoms consistent with hypersexuality during episodes. These included increased masturbation, exposing oneself, obscene language, fondling genitalia, and unwanted sexual advances. These symptoms were also, but more rarely, reported in women and pre-pubescent children.

Several functional imaging studies of the brain of KLS patients during symptomatic periods demonstrated hypoperfusion in the thalamus, hypothalamus, temporal lobes, orbitofrontal and parasagittal frontal lobes, and less commonly basal ganglia [3]. These studies support the fact that KLS pathophysiology involves multiple cortical and sub-cortical regions of the brain rather than the hypothalamus alone.

Currently, there is no effective treatment for KLS, but stimulants, antipsychotics, and mood stabilizers can be used to improve the symptoms of KLS [3].

Klüver and Bucy Syndrome

Klüver and Bucy syndrome (KBS) was first described following bilateral temporal lobectomy, including the uncus and the greater part of the hippocampus in rhesus monkeys [9]. The main symptoms observed were: (1) visual agnosia/psychic blindness, an inability to recognize objects by sight, (2) hyperorality, a strong tendency to examine all available objects by mouth, (3) hypermetamorphosis, an irrepressible tendency to react and attend to every visual stimulus, (4) marked changes in emotional behavior, especially an absence of fear or expressions of anger, (5) hypersexuality. Since then, there have been about 30 reports of complete or partial Human KBS [10], consecutive to bilateral temporal lobes damage (bilateral temporal lobe resection, encephalitis). Symptoms of hypersexuality frequently encountered were exhibitionism, homosexual and heterosexual advances, and masturbation. The historical aspects and clinical features of human KBS are discussed in detail in another chapter of this book by Doug Lanska.

Hypersexual Disorders in Temporal Lobe Epilepsia

Alteration in sexual behavior has been frequently reported in patients with temporal lobe epilepsia (TLE) [11]. The most common interictal sexual behavior disorder associated with TLE is hyposexuality, defined as a decrease of sexual activity accompanied or not, by erectile or orgasmic dysfunction. In contrast, hypersexuality has been observed as an ictal manifestation of TLE. Such seizure can involve erotic feelings that may be accompanied by genital sensations or orgasm. Sexual automatism, masturbation, and exhibitionism have also been reported [12].

Hypersexual Disorders in Dementia

Neurodegenerative diseases, especially frontotemporal and Alzheimer dementia, are very often associated with neuropsychiatric behavior such as agitation, apathy, anxiety, delusions, sleep disorders, and disinhibition. Many authors have tried to classify these neurobehavioral symptoms in different clusters [13]: (1) "psychosis" cluster, including hallucinations and delusion, (2) "affective" cluster, including apathy, depression, and anxiety, and (3) "hyperactive cluster," including aggressiveness, disinhibition, and aberrant motor behavior. Other less reported neuropsychiatric manifestation of dementia is hypersexuality. Hypersexuality, also called "inappropriate sexual behavior," "improper sexual behavior," or "sexually disinhibited behavior" according to authors, include sexual comments, and extreme sexual behaviors such as public masturbation, exhibitionism, sexual advances to other residents. Hypersexuality generally includes the affective or hyperactive clusters as well as eating and sleep disorders. Although these manifestations have been reported rarely, they cause significant alteration in the quality of life and an immense distress to patients and their caregivers.

The prevalence of hypersexuality in demented patients range between 2 and 30%, according to different studies [13]. Women and men had almost equal frequency of sexually disinhibited behaviors (7 and 8%, respectively). In contrast, men showed mainly physical and women verbal sexual behaviors.

Hypersexuality may be regarded as a part of disinhibited behavior or as an independent neuropsychiatric symptom. More recently, hypersexuality in dementia has been considered as an abnormal response to primary reward stimuli, such as food and intoxicants. Perry et al. [14] identified that low volume of subcortical reward-related structures, especially right ventral putamen and pallidum were associated with increased pursuit of primary rewards including hypersexuality.

Unfortunately, none of the sexual assessment instruments in the literature focus on hypersexual behavior in the cognitively impaired elderly population. The assessment of hypersexuality in demented patients is based on interviews carried out with caregivers. Therapeutic options include both non-pharmacological and pharmacological treatments. Non-pharmacological treatments include cognitive/emotion-oriented interventions, sensory stimulation interventions, behavior management techniques, and psychosocial activities. The treatment option includes antidepressants, antipsychotics, anti-epileptics, and in some cases, hormonal therapies [13].

Hypersexuality and Paraphilia in Parkinson Disease

Parkinson disease (PD) is now recognized as a neuropsychiatric disease characterized by both motor and non-motor manifestations. Although behavioral disturbances are important predictors of quality of life in PD patients, these symptoms are unrecognized and undertreated [15]. Behavioral symptoms in PD patients are grouped under the name of impulse control behaviors (ICB) [16]. The ICBs consist of 4 impulse control disorders (ICDs): pathological gambling, compulsive shopping, hyperphagia, and hypersexuality, associated with dopamine dysregulation syndrome in which patients take excessive amount of medication (dopamine). Hypersexuality was the first ICD reported in the literature and can be defined as "a preoccupation with sexual gratification outside the accepted social and personal bounds despite the harm to may be incurred" [17]. Men were more likely than women to be diagnosed with compulsive sexual behaviors [18]. Dopaminergic agonists use and previous history of ICD prior to PD onset were predictors of an active ICD [19].

Hypersexual behaviors encompass compulsive pornography, excessive masturbation, increased libido, extramarital relationships. Paraphilic disorders such as exhibitionism, transvestism, zoophilia, voyeurism, and pedophilia were also rarely reported. Hypersexuality and paraphilia were commonly reported in association with other ICDs [17].

There is a strong association between hypersexuality, other ICD, and dopamine agonist use. A possible explanation is that dopamine agonists had a higher selective affinity for D3 receptors, which are abundant in the ventral striatum and the meso-corticolimbic pathway, a region associated with behavioral addictions and substance abuse disorders [20].

The Parkinson's Disease-Sexual Addiction Screening Test is a short and reliable measure of hypersexuality that was developed and validated in 2013 to be used in everyday practice in patients with PD as a screening instrument for multidimensional aspects of hypersexuality [21].

The pharmacological approach in PD patients experiencing hypersexuality in the context of ICD, consist of reduction, discontinuation or switching to dopaminergic agonists. More recent studies highlighted the effect of STN DBS on hypersexuality [17].

Conclusion

Lesion studies reported here illustrate key subcortical and cortical brain regions that determine human sexual behavior. The subcortical regions comprise the hypothalamus, mediating neuroendocrine, and autonomic aspects of sexual drive and basal ganglia. The cortical regions comprise the frontal lobes mediating the motor components of sexual behavior and the control of sexual response and the temporal lobes implicated in sexual orientation, sexual drive and disorders of sexual function. Recent functional neuroimaging studies illustrate the involvement of the neural network in human sexual behavior. The role of the reward system has been specially highlighted.

References

1 Jarvie HF: Frontal lobe wounds causing disinhibition; a study of six cases. J Neurol Neurosurg Psychiatry 1954;17:14–32.

2 Miller BL, Cummings JL, McIntyre H, Ebers G, Grode M: Hypersexuality or altered sexual preference following brain injury. J Neurol Neurosurg Psychiatry 1986;49:867–873.

3 Miglis MG, Guilleminault C: Kleine-Levin syndrome: a review. Nat Sci Sleep 2014;6:19–26.
4 Kleine W: Periodische schlafsucht. Monats Psychiatr Neurol 1925;57:285–320.
5 Levin M: Periodic somnolence and morbid hunger: a new syndrome. Brain 1936;59:494–504.
6 Critchley M, Hoffman HL: The Syndrome of Periodic Somnolence and Morbid Hunger (Kleine-Levin syndrome). Br Med J 1942;1:137–139.
7 Arnulf I, Lin L, Gadoth N, et al: Kleine-Levin syndrome: a systematic study of 108 patients. Ann Neurol 2008;63:482–493.
8 Arnulf I, Zeitzer JM, File J, Farber N, Mignot E: Kleine-Levin syndrome: a systematic review of 186 cases in the literature. Brain 2005;128(pt 12):2763–2776.
9 Neylan TC, Klüver H, Bucy PC: Temporal lobe and behavior: Klüver and Bucy's classic preliminary analysis of functions of the temporal lobes in monkeys. J Neuropsychiatr 1997;9:606–620.
10 Lilly R, Cummings JL, Benson DF, Frankel M: The human Klüver-Bucy syndrome. Neurology 1983;33: 1141–1145.
11 Baird AD, Wilson SJ, Bladin PF, Saling MM, Reutens DC: Neurological control of human sexual behaviour: insights from lesion studies. J Neurol Neurosurg Psychiatry 2007;78:1042–1049.
12 Freemon FR, Nevis AH: Temporal lobe sexual seizures. Neurology 1969;19:87–90.
13 Torrisi M, Cacciola A, Marra A, De Luca R, Bramanti P, Calabrò RS: Inappropriate behaviors and hypersexuality in individuals with dementia: an overview of a neglected issue. Geriatr Gerontol Int 2017;17: 865–874.
14 Perry DC, Sturm VE, Seeley WW, Miller BL, Kramer JH, Rosen HJ: Anatomical correlates of reward-seeking behaviours in behavioural variant frontotemporal dementia. Brain 2014;137(pt 6):1621–1626.
15 Phu AL, Xu Z, Brakoulias V, et al: Effect of impulse control disorders on disability and quality of life in Parkinson's disease patients. J Clin Neurosci 2014; 21:63–66.
16 Zurowski M, O'Brien JD: Developments in impulse control behaviours of Parkinson's disease. Curr Opin Neurol 2015;28:387–392.
17 Nakum S, Cavanna AE: The prevalence and clinical characteristics of hypersexuality in patients with Parkinson's disease following dopaminergic therapy: A systematic literature review. Parkinsonism Relat Disord 2016;25:10–16.
18 Weintraub D, Koester J, Potenza MN, et al: Impulse control disorders in Parkinson disease: a cross-sectional study of 3090 patients. Arch Neurol 2010;67: 589–595.
19 Weintraub D, David AS, Evans AH, Grant JE, Stacy M: Clinical spectrum of impulse control disorders in Parkinson's disease. Mov Disord 2015;30:121–127.
20 Gurevich EV, Joyce JN: Distribution of dopamine D3 receptor expressing neurons in the human forebrain: comparison with D2 receptor expressing neurons. Neuropsychopharmacology 1999;20:60–80.
21 Pereira B, Llorca PM, Durif F, et al: Screening hypersexuality in Parkinson's disease in everyday practice. Parkinsonism Relat Disord 2013;19:242–246.

M. Béreau, MD
Department of Neurology, CHRU Besançon
3 boulevard Alexandre Fleming
25030 Besançon Cedex (France)
E-Mail mbereau@chu-besancon.fr

Bogousslavsky J (ed): Neurologic-Psychiatric Syndromes in Focus. Part I – From Neurology to Psychiatry.
Front Neurol Neurosci. Basel, Karger, 2018, vol 41, pp 77–89 (DOI: 10.1159/000475721)

The Klüver-Bucy Syndrome

Douglas J. Lanska[a, b]

[a]VA Medical Center, Great Lakes VA Healthcare System, Tomah, WI, and [b]Department of Neurology, University of Wisconsin School of Medicine and Public Health, Madison, WI, USA

Abstract

In 1937, Heinrich Klüver and Paul Bucy described a dramatic behavioral syndrome in monkeys after bilateral temporal lobectomy. The full Klüver-Bucy syndrome (KBS) – hyperorality, placidity, hypermetamorphosis, dietary changes, altered sexual behavior, and visual agnosia – is evident within 3 weeks following operation. Some KBS features (i.e., hyperorality, placidity, hypermetamorphosis) persist indefinitely, whereas others gradually resolve over several years. Klüver and Bucy were initially unaware of an earlier report of KBS by Sanger Brown and Edward Schäfer in 1888. Human cases were recognized in the 1950s, as surgeons employed bilateral temporal lobectomies to treat seizures. Various attempts were made to localize the component features to specific areas of the temporal lobe, with mixed success. Bilateral ventral temporal ablations and bilateral temporal lobectomies produced marked impairment in visual discrimination, whereas lateral resections or unilateral lesions did not. Discrete bilateral lesions of the lateral amygdaloid nucleus produced a permanent "hypersexed state." By the 1970s, it was clear that the major symptoms of KBS are produced by destroying either the temporal neocortex or the amygdala bilaterally. KBS is now thought to be caused by disturbances of temporal portions of limbic networks that interface with multiple cortical and subcortical circuits to modulate emotional behavior and affect. The clinical features of KBS in man are similar to those in monkeys, but the full syndrome is rarely seen, probably because the anterior temporal lobe dysfunction is usually less severe than that following total temporal lobe ablation in monkeys. Human KBS does not occur in isolation, but is typically part of a complex behavioral syndrome that almost always includes amnesia and aphasia, and that may also include dementia and seizures. The treatment of KBS is difficult and often unsatisfactory.

Introduction and History

In 1937, German-born American psychologist Heinrich Klüver (1897–1979) and American neurosurgeon and neuropathologist Paul Clancy Bucy (1904–1992) described a dramatic behavioral syndrome in Rhesus monkeys that had undergone bilateral temporal lobectomy [1–13]. This was an unanticipated consequence of Klüver's studies of the reactions of humans and animals to mescaline, a naturally occurring psychedelic alkaloid similar in its effects to LSD.

In an obituary of Klüver, fellow psychologist William A. Hunt (1903–1986) recounted how Klüver became bored after a few days away from his laboratory while on vacation on a New Hampshire farm:

> [Klüver] began investigating the effects of mescal on the farmer's cow. He overestimated the ameliorating effects of body weight on dosage size and the cow died. Klüver confessed his guilt and reimbursed the farmer, but as Klüver said, "He took it unpleasantly." Klüver also used himself as a subject and consequently suffered an attack of mescal poisoning that left him seriously ill for a while [11, p 160].

As noted in a later biographical memoir, while Klüver was "at the University of Minnesota around 1924, he ingested mescal buttons and compulsively documented the nature of his own experiences during intoxicated states" [13]. Klüver's later work with mescaline produced behavioral manifestations in monkeys that suggested to him that this drug might act on the temporal lobe:

> Our interest in temporal lobe functions was aroused by the discovery of one of us (Klüver) that the injection of mescaline or chemically related substances into monkeys produces peculiar chewing and licking movements as well as convulsions, in other words, symptoms resembling those found in the "uncinate group of fits" described [in 1899] by [English neurologist John] Hughlings Jackson [1835–1911] and [Scottish neurologist James Purves] Stewart [1869–1949]. It was thought desirable, therefore, to remove the temporal lobes, including the uncus [3, pp 989–990].

On this basis, Klüver induced Bucy to perform staged bilateral temporal lobe resections on monkeys to assess whether the effects of mescaline would be ameliorated. On December 7, 1936, Bucy removed most of the left temporal lobe of an aggressive adult female Rhesus monkey named "Aurora" [7, 10, 13]. As Bucy later recounted, the following morning Klüver called him on the telephone and abruptly demanded to know, "What did you do to my monkey?" [10]. Bucy hurried to the office and observed that the once-aggressive monkey had become "tame," a behavioral change that was even more pronounced after Bucy removed the opposite temporal lobe in a subsequent operation on January 25, 1937 [7, 10, 13].

The initial report by Klüver and Bucy in April 1937, presented at the annual meeting of the American Physiological Society in Memphis, Tennessee, described the effects of sequential staged bilateral temporal lobectomy in an adult Rhesus monkey:

> The animal does not exhibit the reactions generally associated with anger and fear. It approaches humans and animals, animate as well as inanimate objects without hesitation and although there are no motor defects, tends to examine them by mouth rather than by the use of hands. There is a general slowing down of movements; the quick, jerky movements characteristic of the normal Rhesus monkey have almost entirely disappeared [1, p 352].

Although the monkey had no impairment in visual acuity or in the ability to visually localize the positions of objects, it seemed unable to recognize objects by sight:

Table 1. Klüver-Bucy syndrome in monkeys

Permanent manifestations
1 Hyperorality (marked oral examination of objects with licking, sucking, chewing movements, and placing of non-food objects in the mouth)
2 Placidity
3 Hypermetamorphosis (constant manual exploration and inappropriate attention to new stimuli)
Temporary manifestations
4 Dietary changes (hyperphagia, pica, coprophagia)
5 Altered sexual behavior (autosexual, heterosexual, homosexual)
6 Sensory agnosias ("psychic blindness")

> The hungry animal, if confronted with a variety of objects, will, for example, indiscriminately pick up [various objects, including uncharacteristically a live snake]. Each object is transferred to the mouth and then discarded if not edible. ... These symptoms of what appears to be "psychic blindness" are not present in four other monkeys ... in which only one temporal lobe has been removed [1, p 353].

As Klüver and Bucy subsequently elaborated, the full Klüver-Bucy syndrome (KBS) – hyperorality, placidity, hypermetamorphosis, dietary changes, altered sexual behavior, and visual agnosia (Table 1) – is evident within 2–3 weeks following operation [3, 5, 6]. Hyperorality was manifest by a marked tendency to place non-food objects in the mouth, and to examine objects orally (e.g., by licking, sucking, biting, or chewing). Hypermetamorphosis referred to constant manual exploration and inappropriate attention to new stimuli, characterized by an immediate motor response upon the visual presentation of an object, regardless of its history or reward value. The term "hypermetamorphosis" had been coined in 1859 by Breslau psychiatrist Heinrich Wilhelm Neumann (1814–1884), and then adopted and propounded by his assistant, German neuropsychiatrist Carl Wernicke (1848–1905), whose later monograph, *Grundriss der Psychiatrie in klinischen Vorlesungen* (*Outline of Psychiatry in Clinical Lectures*, 1906), conveyed the term and concept to Klüver [14]. Dietary changes of KBS included hyperphagia, pica, coprophagia, and ingestion of large quantities of meat (in normally vegetarian monkeys) [3, 5, 6]. Altered sexual behavior was manifest by a marked increase in the frequency and variety (i.e., autosexual, heterosexual, homosexual) of sexual activity, and also in a broadening of stimuli that would precipitate sexual excitation. What Klüver and Bucy initially called "psychic blindness" and later sensory agnosia [1, 3] referred to the apparent inability to recognize and detect the meaning or significance of objects by sight in the absence of any evident impairment in visual acuity or ability. They found that some features of KBS (i.e., hyperorality, placidity, hypermetamorphosis) persist indefinitely, whereas others (i.e., dietary changes, altered sexual behavior, and agnostic disturbances) resolve gradually over several years (Table 1) [6].

Brown and Schäfer observed similar changes in another Rhesus monkey (monkey number 12) in which only the superior temporal gyri were removed bilaterally (Fig. 2) [15].

In 1940, Bucy acknowledged that the "temporal lobe syndrome" (as he and Klüver then referred to KBS) was a phenomenon that had only been observed in nonhuman primates and did not yet have an established human counterpart:

> The temporal lobe still remains the complete enigma. Klüver and I have made only a beginning[,] which indicates that it is of the greatest importance to the animal's mental and emotional economy. However, these preliminary experiments on the monkey must be correlated with observations on man himself before their full significance can be appreciated [16, p 263].

However, human cases of KBS were recognized by the early-to-mid 1950s, as surgeons employed bilateral temporal lobectomies to treat seizures [17].

Disease Pathogenesis

Brown and Schäfer had been primarily interested in the cerebral localization of the special senses, but concluded that, "On localisation of functions the experiment [of bilateral temporal lobe ablation] throws no direct light; what evidence there is being entirely negative" [15, p 312]. Brown and Schäfer excluded significant alterations in any sensory modality as an explanation for KBS, but concluded that it was impossible to determine from animal studies whether there was a loss of the ability to *interpret* sensations and hence to recognize things (i.e., an agnosia):

> Taste, smell, and hearing were unquestionably present, and not only present, but, so far as could be determined, perfectly acute. The animal was repeatedly tested, and was… submitted to special examination by a committee of the Neurological Society appointed for the purpose. Not the slightest doubt was possible as to the continued possession of the senses in this animal, and it is therefore not possible to suppose they are *localised* in the part of the brain which had been bilaterally removed. Whether there was any difference between this animal and normal monkeys in the appreciation of the impressions obtained through those senses is a question regarding which we offer no opinion, nor is it possible, so far as we can see, to form such opinion from experiments upon animals [15, p 326, italics in original].

Instead, Brown and Schäfer suggested that bilateral temporal ablations "produced a temporary general depression of the intellectual faculties, and has reduced the animals, for a time at least, to a mental condition resembling that of an idiot" [15, p 327]. Later that same year, Schäfer again suggested that the observed behavioral changes in monkeys following bilateral temporal lobe damage are a consequence of acquired defects of intelligence and memory.

> The condition was marked by loss of intelligence and memory, so that the animals, although they received and responded to impressions from all these senses, appeared to understand very imperfectly the meaning of such impressions. This was not confined to any one sense, and was most evident with visual impressions. For even objects most familiar to the animals were carefully exam-

ined, felt, smelt, and tasted, exactly as a monkey will examine an entirely strange object, but much more slowly and deliberately. And again, after only a few minutes, on coming across the same object, exactly the same process of examination would be renewed, as if no recollection of it remained. The disposition also became completely altered: both animals exhibited the utmost greediness, losing all the daintiness which characterizes the feeding of monkeys; they also entirely lost their fear of man [18, p 375].

In 1940, Bucy and Klüver acknowledged the priority of Brown and Schäfer in describing KBS, but then dismissed their report because they did not investigate the pathophysiology of the abnormal behaviors:

Unfortunately, however, [Brown and Schäfer] were not impressed by these observations and carried them no further. In fact, they did nothing towards elucidating the mechanisms involved in the behavior they observed. Of course, half a century ago adequate technics for analyzing animal behavior were not available. Our analysis of the alterations in behavior following bilateral temporal lobectomy clearly indicates that the changes in behavior cannot be dismissed by interpreting them as the result of a loss of "memory" and "intelligence" or as a "mental condition resembling that of an idiot," as Brown and Schäfer did [4, p 1145].

Klüver and Bucy tentatively suggested that the monkey had a form of visual agnosia. What Klüver and Bucy initially called "psychic blindness" in 1937 [1], they later linked with several other related terms and concepts, including (1) *Seelenblindheit* (mind blindness), a term coined in 1889 by German physiologist Hermann Munk (1839–1912); (2) "associative mind blindness," a concept introduced in 1890 by German neurologist Heinrich Lissauer (1861–1891) to distinguish a subject's inability to interpret the meaning of what was seen from an inability to consciously perceive and discriminate stimuli (i.e., apperceptive mind blindness); and (3) sensory agnosia [3]. However, in spite of their chosen terminology, Klüver and Bucy held no firm conviction about the underlying pathophysiology.

The type of disturbance [seen in the initial experimental monkey with KBS] seemed to be similar to the "associative mind blindness" of Lissauer. It is true that the diagnosis [of] "agnosia" can be only of practical importance and [so presumably not of theoretical importance as it] merely serves to raise a number of questions. A review of the clinical literature indicates that the more carefully a case is studied the more difficult it may be to decide whether there is really an "agnostic" or merely a "visual" defect, that is, whether the variety of "agnostic" symptoms can be reduced to disturbances of "elementary" or "higher" visual functions. [Russian-Swiss neuropathologist Constantin] von Monakow [1853–1930] and [French psychiatrist Raoul] Mourgue [1886–1950] even raised the question whether the disturbances in the process of recognition, commonly referred to as "agnosia," are the result of an emotional indifference of the subjects, or, in other words, whether "agnostic" symptoms represent merely disturbances in the affective sphere. In view of this, we can consider "psychic blindness" and related symptoms, as described in our first report, merely the starting point for further analysis. [3, pp 979–980].

Beginning in the 1950s, various attempts were made to localize the features of KBS to specific areas of the temporal lobe, with mixed success [19–26]. Bilateral ventral temporal ablations and bilateral temporal lobectomies produced marked impairment in visual discrimination, whereas bilateral lateral temporal resections or any form of unilateral lesion did not [19–23]. Later studies showed that some of the component features of KBS can be localized to definite nuclei of the amygdaloid complex [24, 25]. In particular, discrete bilateral lesions of the lateral amygdaloid nucleus produced a permanent "hypersexed state" after a period of 8–10 weeks following operation, which was intensified if lesions were also placed in the ventral claustrum [24]. By the 1970s, it was clear that the major symptoms of KBS are produced by destroying either the temporal neocortex or the amygdala bilaterally [24, 25]. KBS is now thought to be caused by disturbances of temporal portions of limbic networks that interface with multiple cortical and subcortical circuits to modulate emotional behavior and affect.

Diagnosis

The clinical features of KBS in man are similar to those in monkeys [3, 6, 17, 27–29], but the full syndrome is not often seen, probably because the degree of anterior temporal lobe dysfunction is usually less severe than that following total temporal lobe ablation in monkeys [30]. Human KBS does not occur in isolation, but is typically part of a complex behavioral syndrome that almost always includes amnesia and aphasia, and that may also include dementia and seizures [29]. Some associated features may also reflect brain dysfunction associated with the underlying diseases that extend beyond the anterior temporal lobes. Rarely, unilateral lesions of the amygdala and extra-temporal limbic system have been reported to cause KBS [31, 32].

The most common manifestations of "partial" human KBS are hyperorality and emotional changes, which are among the most persistent features in monkeys [27–30]. Hyperorality, in particular, is a feature of almost all reported human cases, and is felt by some to be a requirement for diagnosis [30]. Bulimia and rapid weight gain occur in some patients, and some ingest inedible non-food items (e.g., shoe polish or feces) [29, 33]. Typically, emotional changes are manifested as blunted affect, apathy, or pet-like compliance (often to non-verbal gestures rather than oral commands), but some may appear depressed, have a labile affect, or less commonly demonstrate agitation or aggression [29, 33]. Hypermetamorphosis is typically manifested by consistent manual exploration of the environment, with subsequent placement of mobile objects into the mouth [29, 33]. Altered sexual behavior may include improper sexually oriented remarks, exhibitionism, attempts at touching the genitals of others, solicitation of sex, masturbation, and attempting sex with inanimate objects. Visual agnosia is most often manifest as prosopagnosia [29].

Although KBS has rarely been recognized in children [34–36], children with KBS can develop all of the behavioral manifestations seen either in adults with bilateral anterior temporal lobe dysfunction [17, 27–29], or in monkeys with bilateral temporal

Table 2. Causes of human Klüver-Bucy syndrome

Acute bitemporal injury or dysfunction	
1	Bilateral temporal lobectomy or amygdalectomy [17, 30]
2	Traumatic brain injury [29, 30, 35, 36]
3	Meningoencephalitis (particularly, herpes simplex encephalitis) [29, 30, 36, 37]
4	Transtentorial herniation
5	Cerebrovascular disease
6	Post-irradiation encephalopathy (especially after nasopharyngeal carcinoma)
7	Metabolic disorders (e.g., anoxic-ischemic encephalopathy, carbon monoxide poisoning [rapid correction of] hyponatremia, and prolonged and severe hypoglycemia)
8	Demyelinating disorders (e.g., acute disseminated encephalomyelitis, multiple sclerosis, osmotic demyelination syndrome, delayed post-anoxic leukoencephalopathy, methotrexate leukoencephalopathy)
9	Epileptic disorders (ictal and post-ictal, and complex partial [psychomotor] status epilepticus)
10	Neoplasms (e.g., gliomas)
11	Developmental/congenital (e.g., bilateral arachnoid cysts)
Progressive neurodegenerative conditions	
1	Frontotemporal dementia (e.g., Pick disease, progressive subcortical gliosis and other chromosome-17-linked dementias) [27–29, 33]
2	Alzheimer disease [27, 29]
3	Huntington chorea
4	Amyotrophic lateral sclerosis
5	Adrenoleukodystrophy
6	Acute intermittent porphyria
7	Neuronal ceroid lipofuscinosis
8	Sanfilippo syndrome (i.e., mucopolysaccharidosis III)
9	Rett syndrome

lobe ablation [3, 6]. Even very young children who have had no environmental learning of sex may have altered sexual behavior, including frequent holding of genitals, intermittent pelvic thrusting, and rubbing of the genitals to inanimate objects upon lying prone [36].

Human KBS can be caused by either acute bitemporal injury or dysfunction, or by progressive neurodegenerative conditions that severely impact the anterior temporal lobe bilaterally (Table 2) [17, 27–30, 32–37]. The causes of acute bitemporal injury or dysfunction, recognized to cause human KBS, include bilateral temporal lobectomy or amygdalectomy [17, 30], traumatic brain injury [29, 30, 35, 36], meningoencephalitis (particularly herpes simplex encephalitis) [29, 30, 36, 37], transtentorial herniation, cerebrovascular disease [32], post-irradiation encephalopathy (especially after nasopharyngeal carcinoma), metabolic disorders (e.g., anoxic-ischemic encephalopathy, carbon monoxide poisoning, [rapid correction of] hyponatremia, and prolonged and severe hypoglycemia), demyelinating disorders (e.g., acute disseminated encephalomyelitis, multiple sclerosis, osmotic demyelination syndrome, delayed post-anoxic leukoencephalopathy, methotrexate leukoencephalopathy), epileptic conditions (i.e., ictal and post-ictal, and complex partial [psychomotor] status epilepticus), neoplasms (e.g., gliomas, paraneoplastic limbic encephalitis), and rarely developmental/congenital disorders (e.g., bilateral arachnoid cysts). Progressive neurodegenerative conditions reported to cause human KBS include frontotemporal dementias (e.g., Pick disease and progressive subcortical gliosis and other chromosome-17-linked dementias) [27–29, 33], Alzheimer disease [27, 29], Huntington chorea, amyotrophic lateral sclerosis, adrenoleukodystrophy, acute intermittent porphyria, neuronal ceroid lipofuscinosis [34], Sanfilippo syndrome (mucopolysaccharidosis III), and Rett syndrome. KBS tends to occur early in frontotemporal dementias and late in Alzheimer's disease [29, 33].

In children, KBS is most often associated with acute bitemporal injury, particularly from trauma, encephalitis, or anoxia [30, 36, 38]. Some children with juvenile neuronal ceroid lipofuscinosis and some girls with Rett syndrome have features of KBS [34]. However, many children with KBS and neurodegenerative conditions have likely been uncritically lumped under terms such as "idiocy" or "autism." KBS and autism commonly occur together in children, and there is considerable overlap of clinical features. Both KBS and autism are associated with impaired social behavior, communication, and imaginative activity, as well as a markedly restricted range of activities and interests. In addition, components of KBS are commonly reported in children with an autistic disorder. This overlap reflects a similar underlying distribution of neural dysfunction, because both disorders result from dysfunction of similar and interconnected bilateral neural structures [3, 6, 17, 27–29]: autism results from bilateral temporal lobe dysfunction, and possibly additional dysfunction of the mesial frontal lobes, the neostriatum, and various nuclear groups in the thalamus.

Treatment and Management

The treatment of KBS is difficult and often unsatisfactory. The behavioral manifestations of KBS often require one-on-one nursing care for extended periods. Behavioral management approaches and a controlled environment may be modestly beneficial in dealing with some of the manifestations of KBS [34]. Carbamazepine has been reported to be beneficial in several patients with KBS, particularly the affective component. Other putative mood-stabilizing agents, such as valproic acid and gabapentin, are worth trying if carbamazepine is either not successful or contraindicated (e.g., because of known allergy). Selective serotonin reuptake inhibitors have been reported to be helpful in patients with KBS following severe traumatic brain injury. A single patient with KBS and dementia reportedly improved with propranolol and leuprolide: propranolol controlled verbal and nonsexual physical aggression, but not sexually aggressive and inappropriate behaviors, whereas these latter symptoms resolved with leuprolide (a potent inhibitor of gonadotropin secretion and consequently of testicular steroidogenesis). Various antipsychotic agents (e.g., haloperidol, haloperidol decanoate, thiothixene) have also been tried with varied and often limited success, but such agents can sometimes be useful in treating associated psychosis and aggression [32].

Conclusions and Future Directions

KBS was discovered twice, by Brown and Schäfer around 1887, and then by Klüver and Bucy in 1936 [1–3, 15]. While both groups recognized the behavioral changes of bilateral temporal lobe ablation as very unusual and even bizarre, Brown and Schäfer dismissed these manifestations as a curiosity because they provided "no direct light" and only "entirely negative" information concerning their primary interest of localizing the cerebral centers for processing different sensory modalities [15, p 312]; Schäfer continued to pursue his original research agenda in neurophysiology of sensory perception, while Brown returned to the United States to pursue a clinical career in neurology and psychiatry, later presenting an influential clinical report of hereditary ataxia. In contrast, Klüver and Bucy, and particularly Klüver, recognized the syndrome as an opportunity to elucidate the role of the temporal lobe in behavior. Klüver abandoned his prior research program on mescaline intoxication, and instead focused on the behavioral manifestations of occipital and temporal lobe ablations in primates and man. These new results fit well into Klüver's psychological orientation to behavior, as he had expressed several years prior to his and Bucy's discovery of KBS:

> [The] question we wish to answer is: What is it that determines the directions and turns of behavior? More specifically, what are the factors which impart certain directions to the animal's behavior in situations in which reactions to sensory stimuli are performed? What are, briefly speaking, the determinants of sensory responses? We are not interested in the fact that there is such a thing as "behavior;" we are interested in the factors responsible for certain kinds of behavior [39, p 332].

As Bucy later wrote of Klüver:

> [It] may come as a surprise that the discovery of the syndrome of bilateral destruction of the temporal lobes came by chance and without prior planning – but not by accident. This discovery was the result of the action of a well-prepared, active, alert mind, which perceived the unexpected and recognized its importance [9, p 350].

Although KBS is now thought to result from disturbances of temporal portions of limbic networks that interface with multiple cortical and subcortical circuits to modulate emotional behavior and affect, we still have only a rudimentary understanding of these networks, the specific roles of different temporal lobe structures in behavior and emotion, and how discrete lesions of these structures produce dramatic changes in behavior seen with KBS.

Bogousslavsky J (ed): Neurologic-Psychiatric Syndromes in Focus. Part I – From Neurology to Psychiatry.
Front Neurol Neurosci. Basel, Karger, 2018, vol 41, pp 90–97 (DOI: 10.1159/000475688)

Diogenes Syndrome

Frédéric Assal

Cognitive Neurology Unit, Neurology, Department of Clinical Neuroscience, Geneva University Hospital and Faculty of Medicine, Genève, Switzerland

Abstract

Diogenes syndrome (DS) is not a specific disease but a real neurobehavioral syndrome, characterized by severe domestic squalor, pathological hoarding, lack of insight into the condition, and no need for help. DS can be secondary when associated to psychosis or bipolar disorder, or primary when it occurs as a single entity, usually in the elderly. DS is a clinically complex transnosographic syndrome for which multidimensional approaches need to be considered: medical, psychiatric, neurological, social, scientific, and ethical. Known for more than 40 years mainly by geriatricians, psychiatrists, nurses or social workers and more recently by forensic specialists, the fine grained mechanisms of the syndrome are still incompletely understood. From a neurocognitive standpoint, frontal vulnerability certainly disrupts normal decision-making processes, explaining squalor, pathological hoarding, and lack of insight but we need to better understand the connection between the main symptoms and the neural underpinning of the full syndrome. We should definitely intervene earlier, before patients refuse any help, and when the syndrome is supposedly milder, to improve our clinical knowledge, follow patients prospectively, experiment hypothesis in laboratory settings, and launch randomized controlled trials for treatments. There is hope for future pharmacological and non-pharmacological strategies to alleviate this socially disastrous condition.

Introduction

Dupré in 1925, then Stevens in 1963 first published cases of elderly patients with self-neglect and extreme lack of hygiene or squalor [1, 2]. Severe self-neglect in old age was more precisely described as a syndrome by Macmillan and Shaw [3] in 1966 in 72 patients in Nottingham, UK, and this condition was called senile breakdown. Domestic and personal squalor (respectively on the floor, walls, ceiling, windows, beds, tables and skin, hair, hands, clothes) were its main features and graded according to 5 degrees of severity. Aged around 70 years and over, subjects lived mostly alone (69%) and were socially isolated. Thirty-four subjects (47%) were considered mentally normal, although they had personality traits such as being often stubborn, aloof, aggressive, suspicious, or secretive. The remaining 38 subjects (53%) were psychotic, mostly with late-onset psychosis. Three cases presented with alcoholism and 20 patients were known to be heavy drinkers; 11 patients were diagnosed with depression and one with bipolar disorder; grief was found in 28 participants (39%); 25% of them were of high average intelligence. Mobility was fairly good and only 15% were severely immobilized. Twenty-two patients (30%) refused any form of assistance. Seven patients died within a few days of admission and at one-year follow-up, 36 patients (50%) had died. Squalor together with syllogomania (hoarding of useless rubbish) constituted what Clark et al. [4] called Diogenes syndrome (DS) in 1975. They coined the term in reference to Diogenes the Cynic (412–323 BC), born in Sinope. This Greek philosopher who lived alone in a barrel, deliberately rejected material comfort and social conventions. He kept his need for clothing and food to a minimum, and begged. In fact, the term is only partially correct since Diogenes did not hoard and had a strong desire to demonstrate self-sufficiency without material possessions. All 30 cases described by Clark lived in a state of squalor and extreme self-neglect; their homes would smell badly, subjects were dressed in multiple layers of dirty clothes although the number of individuals with syllogomania was not mentioned. Most of the subjects lived alone and were known to the community authorities. Poverty did not seem to be an issue. High I.Q (mean of 140, range 105–170) was replicated. Personality disorders were not significant; subjects seemed detached, suspicious, aggressive, group-dependent, and with a tendency to distort reality. More recently, alternative names have been proposed such as among others, the messy house syndrome or the Havisham syndrome [5]. The latter may better reflect the syndrome but DS, the first eponym, remains the seminal term for historical reasons and because it was described by creative physicians who wrote a key paper.

Epidemiology

In the seminal paper of Macmillan, the syndrome was uncommon, the incidence being 5 per 10,000 in individuals aged 60 years and older and living alone [3]. DS is underreported since patients do not complain and cases are reported by neighbors, relatives, or social workers. The current incidence of the full syndrome is not well-known. In a retrospective observational French study, there was 1.6 case per 10,000 inhabitants; only 25% patients with the complete syndrome and 75% with a partial one [6]. It is estimated that 1 out of 1,000 persons over 65 years old live in squalor in Australia [7]. Patients with DS tend to be old, with an average age of 79 years, although younger patients have also been described [4]. In a cross-sectional study of 81 cases, 49% were older than 64, 37% between 64 and 45, and 13%

between 44 and 18 years of age; the sex ratio was 72% for females and 28% for males [8]. The mean age of 80 years and sex ratio of 71% for females were found in the French study [6]. The majority of DS occurs in individuals who live alone; rare cases have been described in siblings and married couples [3, 6, 9]; a majority of them do not have children [6]. DS is not specific to a certain profession or socioeconomic status.

Disease Pathogenesis

Macmillan postulated a rejection and hostile attitude towards the outside world in a vulnerable personality without necessarily being associated with psychosis [3]. Clarke attributed a reaction to late life to social, psychological, and economic stress in a certain type of personality [4]. Nevertheless, the association of personality traits and risk of elder self-neglect among a large community-dwelling population of south Chicago was not confirmed, especially neuroticism, extraversion, and rigidity [10]. There is no particular trigger to the condition and it is not clear if solitude is a definite risk factor or a consequence of decision-making processes. Individuals with DS are usually discovered by neighbors, or firemen called, because of extreme filth, stink, proliferation of insects or rats, or fire. They may be brought to the hospital because of severe illnesses, such as pneumonia or accidents. Several authors attributed DS to frontotemporal dementia (FTD), and both conditions actually share similar symptoms [11, 12]. As a matter of fact, hoarding is not rare in dementia, and particularly in FTD [13, 14]. In a sample of 41 FTD patients, hoarding was found in 42–64%, loss of hygiene in 64–92%, loss of emotional insight in 75–9%, and loss of embarrassment in 92–73%, depending on FTD subtype (behavioral variant, either apathetic or disinhibited, and semantic dementia) [15]. Hoarding is not specific to this particular dementia and also found in Alzheimer's disease (AD), representing 36% of 75 patients in a Taiwanese AD cohort and most commonly with a MMSE lower than 10 [16]. In our series of 4 cases with severe DS, and full syndrome, who were consecutively hospitalized, 3 patients met criteria for AD and 1 for vascular dementia [17]. Utilization and imitation behaviors, described by Lhermitte [18], might facilitate DS, but they have not been systematically evaluated in the syndrome. In 6 elderly patients with severe squalor and heterogeneous dementia subtypes, Gregory found severe frontal executive deficits in all cases; surprisingly, theory of mind and emotional processing was preserved; while 5 of them recognized squalor from photographs, more than half did not for their own [19]. In a much larger sample of patients with squalor, 92.8% had frontal executive deficits; 92.8% lacked insight; impulsivity was less common [20]. The authors concluded that there was a necessary dorsolateral involvement but one could argue that 7.2% of cases did not present any executive dysfunction. The same group compared squalor-hoarding versus squalor-only people and found the latter had significantly more cognitive deficits, and mental flexibility impairment was a predictor of squalor only [21]. One could hypothesize progressive extension of brain pathology in the frontal lobe. Anderson studied brain-lesion patients with pathological hoarding that always persisted despite interventions and obvious consequences [22]. When they compared their lesions with other brain-lesion patients without hoarding, they found particular involvement of the medial prefrontal lesions, including the right polar region and the anterior cingulate. Forced collectionism followed bilateral orbitofrontal damage after brain surgery [23]. Both severe hoarding and squalor symptoms manifested after an anterior communicating artery aneurysm rupture that associated with brain hypoperfusion in the bilateral orbitofrontal cortices, basal forebrain, and right ventromedial caudate [24]. Interestingly, these patients showed normal executive tests with the exception of the Iowa Gambling task in the latter case, underlying a disruption of normal decision-making processes or abnormal impulsivity in the prefrontal cortex.

Pathological hoarding, formerly considered a subtype of obsessive-compulsive disorder, has been proposed as a unique entity in DSM-5 [25]. These patients usually do not present with self-neglect and, very importantly, have an earlier age of onset. Some authors proposed hoarding and DS to belong to the extremes of the same spectrum [26]. Decision-making was studied using fMRI in patients with isolated hoarding disorder. Patients exhibited abnormal activity in the anterior cingulate cortex and insula when compared to normal controls and OCD. More interestingly, lower activity was observed in those regions when they had to decide about items that did not belong to them. By contrast, more activity was found in items that did belong to them [27]. In Parkinson's disease, pathological hoarding – usually without squalor – is well known and has been associated to impulsive buying, obsessive-compulsive symptoms, and disease duration, pinpointing to excessive dopaminergic neurotransmission [28]. Let us just mention the role of dopamine and serotonin in impulse control disorders that is clearly beyond the scope of this paper [29]. To sum up, the exact pathogenesis of the full syndrome is only hypothetical, pinpointing to a predominant orbitofrontal/mesiofrontal-anterior cingulate cortex dysfunction modulated by serotoninergic and dopaminergic neurotransmissions, and not necessarily involving classic executive functions processed in dorsolateral prefrontal cortex.

Diagnosis

DS is complex sometimes, but not unequivocally accompanied by neurological and/or psychiatric comorbidities. Some authors introduced the distinction between primary and secondary DS, whereas the latter is related to psychiatric disorder ranging from schizophrenia to affective disorders [30]. Overall, DS in young individuals tends to be associated with psychosis, alcohol-induced disorder (either as separate or co-morbid diagnosis), affective disorder or obsessive-compulsive disorder whereas in the elderly it is more commonly isolated or associated with dementia (FTD or more advanced stage of AD). Neurological and past psychiatric history is, therefore, crucial. In an isolated new case, complete blood screen, cognitive and neuropsychiatric assessment as well as neuroimaging studies are necessary for diagnosis as well as for medical complications of the syndrome. Up to now, there is no consensus on the diagnostic criteria for DS. Halliday et al. [8] proposed that domestic squalor, evidence of self-neglect, living alone, tendency to hoard, and lack of concern for surroundings would be the 5 diagnostic criteria. In his study, only 22% of individuals met all of them. One core criteria (lack of help/assistance from a patient actually needing it from a social and sometimes medical point of view) plus one out of 3 secondary criteria (lack of concern with the environment, with him/herself and/or both) were suggested in 2010 [6]. As mentioned earlier, DS is mainly discovered by the community. In hospital settings, DS patients should be suspected in any patient with squalor or multiple layers of soiled clothing. It should be confirmed by visiting the patient's home. Among various scales, squalor and hoarding can be assessed using the "Environmental Cleanliness and Clutter Scale" developed by Halliday and Snowdon [31] that consists of 10 questions exploring 4 categories (reduced accessibility, accumulation of items of little value, accumulation of refuse or garbage, cleanliness of floors and carpets) graded from 0 to 3, with a satisfactory inter-rater reliability and a high internal consistency, a score of >12 indicating moderate or severe squalor. There is common accumulation of vermin (insects, particularly cockroaches), rats or mice and excrement (human or animal). Abnormal hoarding of animals together with DS has been called Noah syndrome [32]. Cessation of normal skin cleansing may provoke a brown mask of dirt resembling a carapace [33] or skin anomalies, such as eczema or accumulation of keratinous crusts over the trunk and upper extremities and multiples furuncles due to dirt, dust, bacterial, fungal, and parasitic debris [34]. There is a particular absence of shame of self-neglect or anosognosia; patient even reject any well-meant help and usually minimize their aberrant behavior or rationalize when confronted. The diagnosis is important since patients with self-neglect behavior have been shown to have increased morbidity and almost 6 times greater mortality at one year than age-matched individuals [35]. Patients tend to avoid social contact and assistance. A particular DS case was found dead with blood over his genitals and thighs due to hemorrhage from a rectal adenocarcinoma [36]. DS poses ethical questions for social workers about when to intervene and what the most appropriate interventions might be. Social workers/neighbors need to balance individuals' right to autonomy and self-determination against risk to themselves or others. DS has practical applications in forensic medicine [37], causing legal challenges: bodies can be found dead and mummified or partly consumed by dogs, therefore police may suspect a traumatic etiology, an homicide, or an attack by an animal. A case was found lying supine on the floor under the bed surrounded by his own blood [38]. Therefore, a case of DS by proxy has also been described [39].

Treatment and Management

There is no guideline on how to treat patients with DS and due to the absence of randomized controlled trials, there is no approved pharmacological treatment. Treatments frequently depend on associated psychiatric symptoms, such as mania or psychosis when present. Overall, pharmacological and non-pharmacological management is difficult since most patients deny their condition, avoid medical attention, and their compliance to any help and therapy is usually poor. In one DS case, risperidone reduced hoarding at 3 mg/day but caused stiffness, slowing of speech, and thinking [40]. A combination of quetiapine up to 600 mg/day and sodium valproate up to 1,200 mg/day abolished DS symptoms in one FTD patient [41]. Lithium significantly improved another patient with a longstanding DS, but possibly secondary to a manic episode and bipolar disorder [42]. Moving the patient to another accommodation is sometimes mandatory [43]. For most professionals, outpatient treatment through community care should be privileged if there is little risk to the patient or neighbors, and management should be conducted in a very sensitive way otherwise patients return to the same living conditions, with even more resistance to support and follow-up. Behavior therapy-based skills training, which included time ranges allocated to specific daily tasks, such as meals, toileting and bathing, physical exercise, and daily non-structured, and structured recreational activities was apparently successful in one case [44].

Conclusions and/or Future Directions

DS remains a complex and transnosographic neurobehavioral syndrome. The increased life expectancy and higher consecutive number of elderly individuals living alone will in all likelihood mean that our society will be faced with more cases. There is no doubt that DS results from a decision-making deficit underpinned by an orbitofrontal and mediofrontal/anterior cingulate network, partly modulated by serotoninergic and dopaminergic neurotransmission, but we need to better understand the syndrome at different levels. First, we need consensus on the diagnostic criteria. More phenomenological, especially in prodromal cases with DS, and longitudinal data should be obtained. The presence of each symptom should be better assessed to decorticate the links between them. From a cognitive neuroscience point of view, we need to design specific behavioral experiments with decision-making tasks coupled to quantified EEG and fMRI to more precisely uncover the neural correlates of the syndrome and try to modulate it. We could imagine intervening with innovative neuroscience techniques, such as transcranial magnetic stimulation or neurofeedback. Finally, we need randomized controlled trials, comparing pharmacological treatments and behavioral therapy. Since we know social isolation is an important contributing factor, we should intervene at the individual level as early as possible, before chronicization where patients deny their problem and refuse any help. Early interventions from social workers, families, and caregivers when available, and not costly medical ones, might also be preventive and limit harm to both patients and community. Let us hope that the new DSM-5 nosography of hoarding disorders – although mainly centered around younger psychiatric patients – and recent articles in the press will contribute to the public knowledge of this fascinating syndrome and consecutively encourage research.

Further Reading

Apart from MacMillan [3], Clark [4] and Cipriani [5], I would definitely advocate the reader to read the spectacular descriptions and photographs of our colleagues from South America and India [32–34].

References

1 Dupré E: Les mendiants thésauriseurs. Pathologies de l'imagination et de l'émotivité. Paris, Payot 1925, pp 431–444.
2 Stevens R: Self-neglect in the elderly. Br J Geriatr Practice 1963;2:88–91.
3 Macmillan D, Shaw P: Senile breakdown in standards of personal and environmental cleanliness. Br Med J 1966;2:1032–1037.
4 Clark A, Mankikar G, Gray I: Diogenes syndrome. A clinical study of gross neglect in old age. Lancet 1975; 305:366–368.
5 Cipriani G, Lucetti C, Vedovello M, Nuti A: Diogenes syndrome in patients suffering from dementia. Dialogues Clin Neurosci 2012;14:455–460.
6 Monfort J-C, Hugonot-Diener L, Devouche E, Wong C, Péan I: Le syndrome de Diogène et les situations apparentées d'auto-exclusion sociale. Enquête descriptive. Psychol NeuroPsychiatr Vieil 2010;8:141–153.
7 Lee S, LoGiudice D: Phenomenology of squalor, hoarding and self-neglect: an Australian aged care perspective. Intern Med J 2012;42:98–101.
8 Halliday G, Banerjee S, Philpot M, Macdonald A: Community study of people who live in squalor. Lancet 2000;355:882–886.
9 Halliday G, Snowdon J, Simpson B: Re: diogenes syndrome in a pair of siblings. Can J Psychiatry 2005; 50:567.
10 Dong X, Simon M, Wilson R, Beck T, McKinell K, Evans D: Association of personality traits with elder self-neglect in a community-dwelling population. Am J Geriatr Psychiatry 2011;19:743–751.
11 Beauchet O, Imler D, Cadet L, Blanc P, Ramboa P, Girtanner C, Gonthier R: [Diogenes syndrome in the elderly: clinical form or frontal dysfunction? Report of 4 cases]. Rev Med Interne 2002;2:122–131.
12 Orrell MW, Sahakian BJ, Bergmann K: Self-neglect and frontal lobe dysfunction. Br J Psychiatry 1989; 155:101–105.
13 Mendez MF, Shapira JS: The spectrum of recurrent thoughts and behaviors in frontotemporal dementia. CNS Spectr 2008;13:202–208.
14 Perry DC, Whitwell JL, Boeve BF, Pankratz VS, Knopman DS, Petersen RC, Jack CR Jr, Josephs KA: Voxel-based morphometry in patients with obsessive-compulsive behaviors in behavioral variant frontotemporal dementia. Eur J Neurol 2012;19: 911–917.
15 Snowden JS, Hu Q, Rollinson S, Halliwell N, Robinson A, Davidson YS, Momeni P, Baborie A, Griffiths TD, Jaros E, Perry RH, Richardson A, Pickering-Brown SM, Neary D, Mann DM: The most common type of FTLD-FUS (aFTLD-U) is associated with a distinct clinical form of frontotemporal dementia but is not related to mutations in the FUS gene. Acta Neuropathol 2011;122:99–110.
16 Hwang JP, Yang CH, Tsai SJ, Liu KM: Behavioural disturbances in psychiatric inpatients with dementia of the Alzheimer's type in Taiwan. Int J Geriatr Psychiatry 1997;12:902–906.
17 Bruggimann L, Weber K, Michon A, Assal F: Diogenes Syndrome in the Elderly: a behavioral syndrome associated with dementia. Int Psychogeriatrics 2005, Cambridge University Press, New York.

18 Lhermitte F: 'Utilization behaviour' and its relation to lesions of the frontal lobes. Brain 1983;106:237–255.
19 Gregory C, Halliday G, Hodges J, Snowdon J: Living in squalor: neuropsychological function, emotional processing and squalor perception in patients found living in squalor. Int Psychogeriatr 2011;23:724–731.
20 Lee SM, Lewis M, Leighton D, Harris B, Long B, Macfarlane S: Neuropsychological characteristics of people living in squalor. Int Psychogeriatr 2014;26: 837–844.
21 Lee SM, Lewis M, Leighton D, Harris B, Long B, Macfarlane S: A comparison of the neuropsychological profiles of people living in squalor without hoarding to those living in squalor associated with hoarding. Int J Geriatr Psychiatry 2016; DOI: 10.1002/gps.4631.
22 Anderson SW, Damasio H, Damasio AR: A neural basis for collecting behaviour in humans. Brain 2005; 128:201–212.
23 Volle E, Beato R, Levy R, Dubois B: Forced collectionism after orbitofrontal damage. Neurology 2002; 58:488–490.
24 Funayama M, Mimura M, Koshibe Y, Kato Y: Squalor syndrome after focal orbitofrontal damage. Cogn Behav Neurol 2010;23:135–139.
25 American Psychiatric Association: Diagnostic and Statistical Manual of Mental Disorders: DSM 5 2013; American Psychiatric Association, Arlington, VA.
26 Lavigne B, Hamdan M, Faure B, Merveille H, Pareaud M, Tallon E, Bouthier A, Clément JP, Calvet B: Syndrome de Diogène et Hoarding disorder: une même entité? Encéphale 2016;42:421–425.
27 Tolin DF, Stevens MC, Villavicencio AL, Norberg MM, Calhoun VD, Frost RO, Steketee G, Rauch SL, Pearlson GD: Neural mechanisms of decision making in hoarding disorder. Arch Gen Psychiatry 2012; 69:832–841.
28 O'Sullivan SS, Djamshidian A, Evans AH, Loane CM, Lees AJ, Lawrence AD: Excessive hoarding in Parkinson's disease. Mov Disord 2010;25:1026–1033.
29 Rogers RD: The roles of dopamine and serotonin in decision making: evidence from pharmacological experiments in humans. Neuropsychopharmacology 2011;36:114–132.
30 Reyes-Ortiz CA: Diogenes syndrome: the self-neglect elderly. Compr Ther 2001;27:117–121.
31 Halliday G, Snowdon J: The Environmental Cleanliness and Clutter Scale (ECCS). Int Psychogeriatr 2009;21:1041–1050.
32 Saldarriaga-Cantillo A, Rivas Nieto JC: Noah Syndrome: A variant of diogenes syndrome accompanied by animal hoarding practices. J Elder Abuse Negl 2015;27:270–275.
33 Nayak K, Gopinath H, Kini H, Kumar P: Unmasking diogenes syndrome. Indian J Dermatol 2015;60:287.
34 Biswas P, Ganguly A, Bala S, Nag F: Choudhary N, Sen S: Diogenes syndrome: a case report. Case Rep Dermatol Med 2013;2013:595192.
35 Dong X, Simon M, Mendes de Leon C, Fulmer T, Beck T, Hebert L, Dyer C, Paveza G, Evans D: Elder self-neglect and abuse and mortality risk in a community-dwelling population. JAMA 2009;302:517–526.
36 Freeman A, Byard RW: Fatal hemorrhage from an undiagnosed rectal carcinoma in a case of Diogenes syndrome. Forensic Sci Med Pathol 2014;10:16–118.
37 Byard RW, Tsokos M: Forensic issues in cases of Diogenes syndrome. Am J Forensic Med Pathol 2007; 28:177–181.
38 De-Giorgio F, Grassi VM, Chillemi E, Martinotti G: Dead under the bed: a case of Diogenes syndrome? Int J Geriatr Psychiatry 2013;28:548–549.
39 O'Mahony D, Evans JG: Diogenes syndrome by proxy. Br J Psychiatry 1994;164:705–706.
40 Herrán A, Vázquez-Barquero JL: Treatment of Diogenes syndrome with risperidone. Aging Neuropsychol Cognition 1999;6:96–98.
41 Gálvez-Andres A, Blasco-Fontecilla H, Gonzalez-Parra S, de Dios Molina J, Padín JM, Rodriguez RH: Secondary bipolar disorder and Diogenes syndrome in frontotemporal dementia: behavioral improvement with quetiapine and sodium valproate. J Clin Psychopharmacol 2007;27:722–723.
42 Fond G, Jollant F, Abbar M: The need to consider mood disorders, and especially chronic mania, in cases of Diogenes syndrome (squalor syndrome). Int Psychogeriatr 2011;23:505–507.
43 Vostanis P, Dean C: Self neglect in adult life. Br J Psychiatry 1992;161:265–267.
44 Waserman JE, Hategan A, Bourgeois JA: Harnessing neuroplasticity in Diogenes syndrome: a proposed mechanism to explain clinical improvement. Gen Hosp Psychiatry 2014;36:761.e3–e5.

Dr. Frédéric Assal
Service de Neurologie, Département de Neurosciences Cliniques, HUG
Gabrielle Perret Gentil 4
CH–1211 Genève 11 (Switzerland)
E-Mail Frederic.Assal@hcuge.ch

Bogousslavsky J (ed): Neurologic-Psychiatric Syndromes in Focus. Part I – From Neurology to Psychiatry.
Front Neurol Neurosci. Basel, Karger, 2018, vol 41, pp 98–103 (DOI: 10.1159/000475701)

Brueghel Syndrome or Meige Syndrome? Two Sides of a Same Disease

M. Béreau[a] · L. Tatu[b]

[a]Department of Neurology, CHRU Besançon, and [b]Department of Neuromuscular Diseases and Department of Anatomy, CHRU Besançon, University of Franche-Comté, Besançon, France

Abstract

Different eponyms such as "Wood syndrome," Meige syndrome, "Brueghel syndrome," "Blepharospasm plus syndrome" have been used to describe segmental craniocervical dystonias. These facial and/or oromandibular movement disorders are characterized by muscle contractions and spasms involving eyes, facial region, and sometimes pharynx, jaw, floor of the mouth, and tongue. The pathophysiology of craniocervical dystonia is poorly understood, but abnormal plasticity and impaired inhibition are suspected. Injection of botulinum toxin appears to be the best therapeutic option for treating segmental craniocervical dystonia. The objective of this chapter is to depict the history of segmental craniocervical dystonia in order to delineate the phenotypic spectrum of the disorders and to distinguish this entity from other facial and/or oromandibular movement disorders.

Introduction

The eponymic terms *"Meige syndrome"* and *"Brueghel syndrome"* have been used since 1970s to characterize blepharospasm-plus syndrome, defined as a combination of blepharospasm and lower face muscle and/or masticatory muscle dystonia. These multiple and confusing terms led to the description of the segmental craniocervical dystonia spectrum. This anatomically-based classification of dystonia includes blepharospasm, oromandibular dystonia, and blepharospasm-plus syndromes, and also Meige and Brueghel syndromes. In this chapter, we present the history of segmental craniocervical dystonia and discuss the diagnosis, pathophysiology, and treatment of these movement disorders.

History

Horatio Wood (1841–1920), a Philadelphia neurologist, first mentioned blepharospasm and other cranial dystonias in 1887 [1]. However, this movement disorder was described in detail in 1910 by Henry Meige (1866–1940), a French neurologist, who made significant contribution towards the individualization of this clinical entity. Meige depicted ten patients with involuntary eyelid closure and bilateral *"facial convulsions"* [2]. Within *"facial convulsions,"* he identified blepharospasm, another phenotype distinct from hemifacial spasm and facial epileptic seizures. He characterized blepharospasm as bilateral and median facial convulsions that predominate in the orbicularis oculi muscles, in subjects who complained of blindness following complete closure of eyes. Meige highlighted the main clinical features of blepharospasm, especially tonic muscle contractions "blepharotonus" leading to the closure of eyes, and clonic muscle contractions. Interestingly, he emphasized that *"facial convulsions"* were also observed in other facial muscles including frontal muscles, perioral, and perinasal muscles. In one patient, bilateral *"facial convulsions"* were accompanied by contractions of the jaw muscles. These later 2 features have progressively led to the description of the eponymic Meige syndrome.

In 1970s, neurologists rediscovered this clinical entity. Paulson described 3 patients with blepharospasm and oromandibular dystonia as Meige syndrome [3]. Moreover, Altrocchi [4] described 2 patients with isolated oromandibular dystonia and named this condition *"spontaneous orofacial-dyskinesia."* In 1976, Marsden [5] described 39 patients with blepharospasm and oromandibular dystonia. They preferred the eponymous Brueghel syndrome rather than Meige syndrome. They argued that Pieter Brueghel the Elder (ca. 1525–1569), a Flemish Renaissance painter, "clearly recognized the syndrome" in his painting De Gaper depicting a man with eyes closed and mouth wide open (Fig. 1). The authors distinguished this dystonic movement disorder from orofacial drug-induced dyskinesia, and stated that blepharospasm and oromandibular dystonia could occur independently or together. Interestingly, they also defined 2 phenotypes of oromandibular dystonia. In some patients: "The jaw might be forced open and the lips retracted with spasm of platysma and the tongue protruded." In other patients, "the spasms would forcibly close the jaw and the lips would purse like a fish". "These conditions induced marked consequences in both speaking and swallowing" [5].

Despite Peter Brueghel's fascination with normal and pathologic human conditions, an overinterpretation of his *De Gaper* painting is still discussed. Some authors considered that this painting only depicts a yawning man [6].

According to Gilbert, it may be possible to distinguish Brueghel and Meige syndromes [7]. The main difference between these 2 syndromes is that blepharospasm appears to be the essential and sometimes the only feature of Meige syndrome whereas the main sign in Brueghel syndrome is dystonic opened jaw. He pointed out that these 2 syndromes had been frequently confused in the literature. Finally, he suggest-

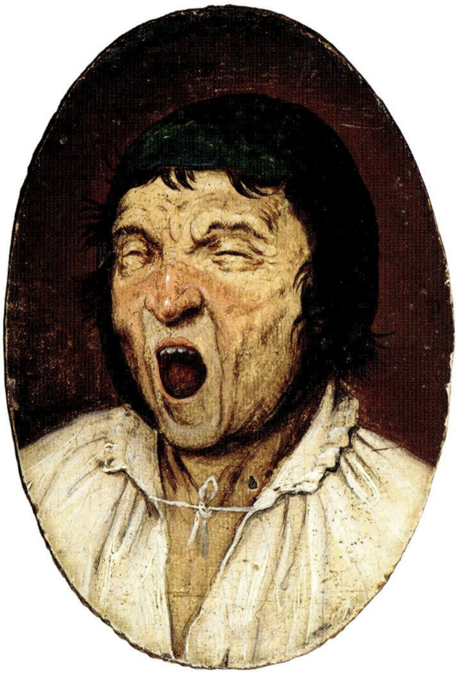

Fig. 1. De Gaper or Yawning Man. Pieter Brueghel the Elder (1527–1569). Musées Royaux des Beaux-Arts Bruxelles. © Royal Museums of Fine Arts of Belgium, Brussels / photo: J. Geleyns – Art Photography.

ed that Meige and Brueghel syndromes should be separated based on different pathophysiological mechanisms involving the facial nerve in Meige syndrome and the motor trigeminal nerve in Brueghel syndrome.

More recently in 2011, Ledoux proposed to drop these *"confusing eponymic terms"* for the craniocervical region and developed an anatomically based classification of dystonia [8]. Thus, the term segmental craniocervical dystonia appears to be more accurate than Meige or Brueghel syndromes in patients with blepharospasm-plus syndrome. This classification was consistent with the consensus update concerning classification of dystonia published in 2013 [9].

Epidemiology

There is a wide variability in the prevalence estimates of segmental craniocervical dystonia. However, prevalence for all anatomical patterns of segmental dystonia has been estimated at 32 per million [10]. Age appears to be an independent risk factor in the development of segmental craniocervical dystonia with an average age of onset in the sixth decade. Segmental craniocervical dystonias were also more common in females than males (sex ratio of 2:1) [11]. Associated movement disorders have also been frequently reported in segmental craniocervical patients, especially essential tremor [12], Parkinson disease, and atypical parkinsonism [13].

Disease Pathogenesis

The pathophysiology of segmental craniocervical dystonia and other focal dystonia remains a topic of debate. Numerous brain regions and neural networks, especially sensorimotor cortex, brain stem, and basal ganglia have been suspected to be involved [14]. Neurophysiological studies using paired-pulse transcranial magnetic stimulation of the contralateral primary motor area have shown a reduction of intracortical inhibition in patients with focal dystonia [15]. This reduction would explain increased excitability of motor area and followed by the overflow phenomenon. Moreover, the cortical silent period, a marker of cortical motor excitability that can also be studied by transcranial magnetic stimulation, was reduced in affected muscles of patients with cranial, cervical, and hand dystonia. Interestingly, in patients with blepharospasm, the silent period was also shortened in perioral muscles [16]. fMRI studies confirm overactivity of the primary somatosensory cortex and the caudal supplementary motor area in patients with cranial dystonia [17].

Current knowledge attributes a key role to basal ganglia in the pathophysiology of focal dystonia. Neuropathological studies and case reports have emphasized the link between Parkinson disease and blepharospasm, Meige syndrome, and other cranial dystonia. Mark et al. [18] observed that neuropathological case series of Meige syndrome frequently showed Lewis bodies and postulated that in some cases Meige syndrome should be included in the spectrum of Lewy bodies disease. Other studies highlighted that cranial dystonia patients were more likely to develop Parkinson disease, thus suggesting a common basal ganglia dysfunction in the pathophysiology of both disorders [19]. Wicki et al. [20] reported Brueghel syndrome (facial dystonia with wide opening of the mouth) as a manifestation of HIV encephalopathy in one patient. Brain MRI showed abnormalities in the bilateral lenticular nucleus. Interestingly, Brueghel syndrome and MRI abnormalities improved dramatically a few days after antiretroviral therapy was initiated. Morphological neuroimaging studies have also supported the role of basal ganglia in the pathophysiology of cranial dystonia. Volumetric imaging studies showed significantly larger putamina in patients with cranial dystonia [21]. Moreover, transcranial sonography study showed hyperechogenic lesions in the lenticular nucleus in facial dystonia patients [22].

Diagnosis

In the current classification of movement disorders, segmental craniocervical dystonia spectrum encompasses isolated blepharospasm, isolated oromandibular dystonia, and blepharospasm-plus syndrome, defined as a combination of blepharospasm, and other cranial or/and cervical dystonia [8]. Currently, Meige and Brueghel syndromes are included in blepharospasm-plus syndrome. Blepharospasm is the most common manifestation of craniocervical dystonia and can be present in various phenotypic clinical forms [23]. The most characteristic one is the tonic form characterized by prolonged spasm of eye closure called tonic spasms. The clonic form is defined by recurrent abnormal contractions of orbicularis oculi muscles. Blepharospasm may spread to the lower facial and masticatory muscles involved in chewing, jaw opening, and jaw closing leading to the blepharospasm-plus syndrome. The probability of extension to the lower facial muscles is higher within the initial five years [23].

The diagnostic approaches of segmental craniocervical dystonia consist in characterizing the movement disorder and ruling out a neurodegenerative or treatable etiology. Electromyographic patterns are sometimes helpful in specifying facial abnormal movements showing muscular hyperactivity or spasms. Brain MRI is also useful in ruling out secondary dystonia (spinocerebellar ataxia, progressive supranuclear palsy…) and bilateral hemifacial spasms due to neurovascular conflicts. Medications which block dopamine receptors in the brain should also be considered [23].

Treatment and Management

Many oral medications have been used in treating segmental craniocervical dystonia, including anticholinergics, benzodiazepines, and atypical antipsychotics [8]. However, there is no evidence of the effectiveness of these medications. Nevertheless, anticholinergics and clonazepam, although with numerous side effects, would improve segmental craniocervical dystonia, especially blepharospasm [24].

Botulinum toxin injections are the most appropriate treatment for segmental craniocervical dystonia. Several studies have corroborated dramatic improvement with injections of botulinum toxin in blepharospasm patients [12]. Blepharospasm showed better response to injections compared to oromandibular and lower face dystonia. Successful treatment with botulinum toxin requires an accurate knowledge of craniocervical muscles anatomy. In case of oromandibular dystonia, electromyographic guidance is a valuable tool to better targeting of involved muscles. Adverse events, especially weakness of nearby muscles, are transient and reversible.

More recently, deep brain stimulation of globus pallidus interna has emerged as an alternative therapeutic option in patients with intractable craniocervical dystonia [25].

Conclusion

Although Brueghel syndrome is one of the only artistic attribution of a neurologic disorder, this eponymic term as well as Meige syndrome should be avoided in favor of segmental craniocervical dystonia, an anatomically based classification of focal dystonia.

References

1 Wood HC: A Treatise on Therapeutics, Comprsising Materia Medica and Toxicology, with Special Reference to the Application of Physiological Action of Drugs to Clinical Medecine. Philadelphia, Lippincott, 1874.

2 Meige H: Les convulsions de la face: une forme clinique de convulsion faciale, bilaterale et mediane. Rev Neurol (Paris) 1910;10:437–443.

3 Paulson GW: Meige's syndrome. Dyskinesia of the eyelids and facial muscles. Geriatrics 1972;27:69–73.

4 Altrocchi PH: Spontaneous oral-facial dyskinesia. Arch Neurol 1972;26:506–512.

5 Marsden CD: Blepharospasm-oromandibular dystonia syndrome (Brueghel's syndrome). A variant of adult-onset torsion dystonia? J Neurol Neurosurg Psychiatry 1976;39:1204–1209.

6 Garcia-Ruiz PJ, Slawek J, Sitek EJ, Martinez Castrillo JC: Art and dystonia. J Neurol Sci 2015;356:49–54.

7 Gilbert GJ: Brueghel syndrome: its distinction from Meige syndrome. Neurology 1996;46:1767–1769.

8 LeDoux MS: Meige syndrome: what's in a name? Parkinsonism Relat Disord 2009;15:483–489.

9 Albanese A, Bhatia K, Bressman SB, et al: Phenomenology and classification of dystonia: a consensus update. Mov Disord 2013;28:863–873.

10 Epidemiological Study of Dystonia in Europe (ESDE) Collaborative Group: A prevalence study of primary dystonia in eight European countries. J Neurol 2000;247:787–792.

11 Grandas F, Elston J, Quinn N, Marsden CD: Blepharospasm: a review of 264 patients. J Neurol Neurosurg Psychiatry 1988;51:767–772.

12 Lou JS, Jankovic J: Essential tremor: clinical correlates in 350 patients. Neurology 1991;41(2 pt 1):234–238.

13 Rana AQ, Kabir A, Dogu O, Patel A, Khondker S: Prevalence of blepharospasm and apraxia of eyelid opening in patients with parkinsonism, cervical dystonia and essential tremor. Eur Neurol 2012;68:318–321.

14 Defazio G, Berardelli A, Hallett M: Do primary adult-onset focal dystonias share aetiological factors? Brain 2007;130(pt 5):1183–1193.

15 Sommer M, Ruge D, Tergau F, Beuche W, Altenmüller E, Paulus W: Intracortical excitability in the hand motor representation in hand dystonia and blepharospasm. Mov Disord 2002;17:1017–1025.

16 Currà A, Romaniello A, Berardelli A, Cruccu G, Manfredi M: Shortened cortical silent period in facial muscles of patients with cranial dystonia. Neurology 2000;54:130–135.

17 Dresel C, Haslinger B, Castrop F, Wohlschlaeger AM, Ceballos-Baumann AO: Silent event-related fMRI reveals deficient motor and enhanced somatosensory activation in orofacial dystonia. Brain 2006;129(pt 1):36–46.

18 Mark MH, Sage JI, Dickson DW, et al: Meige syndrome in the spectrum of Lewy body disease. Neurology 1994;44:1432–1436.

19 Micheli F, Scorticati MC, Folgar S, Gatto E: Development of Parkinson's disease in patients with blepharospasm. Mov Disord 2004;19:1069–1072.

20 Wicki J, Germanier Y, Sztajzel R, Burkhard PR: Brueghel syndrome as a new manifestation of HIV encephalopathy. Eur Neurol 2008;60:107–108.

21 Black KJ, Ongür D, Perlmutter JS: Putamen volume in idiopathic focal dystonia. Neurology 1998;51:819–824.

22 Becker G, Naumann M, Scheubeck M, et al: Comparison of transcranial sonography, magnetic resonance imaging, and single photon emission computed tomography findings in idiopathic spasmodic torticollis. Mov Disord 1997;12:79–88.

23 Pandey S, Sharma S: Meige's syndrome: history, epidemiology, clinical features, pathogenesis and treatment. J Neurol Sci 2017;372:162–170.

24 Hípola D, Mateo D, Giménez-Roldán S: Meige's syndrome: acute and chronic responses to clonazepan and anticholinergics. Eur Neurol 1984;23:474–478.

25 Houser M, Waltz T: Meige syndrome and pallidal deep brain stimulation. Mov Disord 2005;20:1203–1205.

M. Béreau, MD
Department of Neurology, CHRU Besançon
3 Boulevard Alexandre Fleming
FR–25030 Besançon Cedex (France)
E-Mail mbereau@chru-besancon.fr

Bogousslavsky J (ed): Neurologic-Psychiatric Syndromes in Focus. Part I – From Neurology to Psychiatry.
Front Neurol Neurosci. Basel, Karger, 2018, vol 41, pp 104–116 (DOI: 10.1159/000478914)

REM Sleep Behavior Disorder
A Unique Window into Dreaming, the Violent Brain and Early Mechanisms of Neurodegeneration

Claudio L. Bassetti · Panagiotis Bargiotas

Neurology Department, Inselspital, Bern University Hospital, Bern, Switzerland

Abstract

Rapid eye movement sleep behavior disorder (RBD) is a brain disorder, characterized by the dream enactment during rapid eye movement (REM) sleep due to a lack of physiologic muscle atonia and increased muscle twitching. Schenk was the first to describe this disorder in 1986; however, few authors reported in the 1970–1980s loss of physiological muscle atonia combined with dream enactment in the course of brainstem disorders and as a consequence of alcoholism and antidepressant treatment. RBD affects less than 1% of the adult population, but can be found in up to 25–50% of neurodegenerative disorders including Parkinson's disease, multisystem atrophy, and dementia with Lewy body. In the last decade, many studies provided evidence that RBD precedes parkinsonian motor signs by several years, suggesting that RBD should no longer be considered a complication but a part of the prodromal phase of these diseases. Etiologically, primary (idiopathic RBD) and several secondary forms in addition to neurodegeneration (related to focal brainstem damage, narcolepsy, autoimmune disorders, and drugs) are known. Pathophysiologically, brainstem and supratentorial mechanisms involving glutamatergic, glycinergic, and GABA-ergic neurotransmission have been implicated. Recently, an animal model of RBD has been described. Clinical features consist of characteristic nocturnal behaviors, but also daytime symptoms including excessive sleepiness and cognitive alterations. The diagnosis of RBD is made according to international diagnostic criteria, based on medical history, and video-polysomnographic features. Current treatment strategies include actions which ensure a safe sleep environment, the avoidance of triggering/exacerbating factors and if necessary pharmacological (mainly clonazepam and melatonin) and non-pharmacological (e.g., behavioral measures) interventions. Future research should clarify the exact sleep-wake characteristics of RBD (also beyond REM sleep) and their evolution over time, the contribution of brainstem but also supratentorial mechanisms to its pathophysiology, and the (early?) diagnostic and (causative?) treatment consequences of RBD in the context of neurodegeneration.

Introduction/History

Rapid eye movement sleep behavior disorder (RBD) is characterized by an abnormal behavior arising from rapid eye movement (REM) sleep, which is accompanied by (oft frightening) vivid dreaming [1, 2].

Physiologically, in REM sleep the sleeping person is mentally active and dreaming, while the skeletal muscles are paralyzed. In RBD however, this atonia is disturbed, which allows the patient to "act out his dreams," exhibiting a variety of motor activities. Typically, RBD occurs repeatedly in the second part of the night.

In 1965, Jouvet and Delorme reported for the first time on the persistent loss of physiological muscle atonia and new onset of hallucinatory behaviors during REM sleep in cats with symmetrical dorsolateral pontine tegmental lesions [3]. Schenck was the first to formally describe RBD in 1986; however, before this formal description few authors reported cases of physiological muscle atonia loss combined with dream enactment [4]. The most characteristic cases are those reported during the early 1970s by Passouant et al. [5], Tachibana et al. [6], and De Barros et al. [7], where authors described the loss of physiological muscle atonia combined with dream enactment as a consequence of antidepressant treatment, alcoholism, and in the course of brainstem disorders.

Interestingly, the earliest references to dream enacting behavior can be traced in non-scientific texts and in literature much earlier than these first reports, and the formal description by Schenk et al. Miguel Cervantes in his famous "Don Quixote" (1615) included masterful descriptions of several sleep disorders including a scene that has been interpreted as dream enactment [8]. In this incidence, Don Quixote's sleep behavior is altered; he is shouting and attacking some wineskins while dreaming that he is fighting a giant (Fig. 1). In addition, 35 years before the first description of RBD we meet a cinematic presentation of the disorder. In 1950 Disney film "Cinderella," the dog Bruno is sleeping in the kitchen showing a typical dream enactment involving chasing Cinderella's cat Lucifer. When Cinderella wakes him up, Bruno seems to be relaxed and he is able to recall the dream.

Epidemiology

Large epidemiological studies on the prevalence of RBD are lacking. The disease affects less than 1% of the general adult population and 2–8% of the older adult population [9]. However, RBD can be commonly found in the context of neurodegenerative disorders, such as Parkinson's disease (PD), multisystem atrophy, and dementia with Lewy body [10–12] but also in narcolepsy [13] and rarely also in the context of a non-REM/REM overlap parasomnia and its extreme form of a wake-sleep state breakdown (status dissociatus) [14, 15]. In a PD cohort, among 120 patients, 37% had

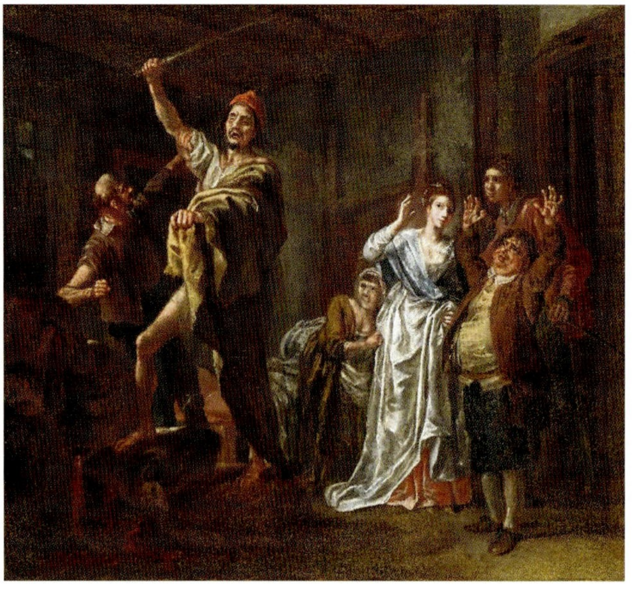

Fig. 1. Francis Hayman (1708–1776): Don Quixote's battle with wine skins. "And in his right hand he held his unsheathed sword, with which he was slashing about on all sides, uttering exclamations as if he were actually fighting some giant: and the best of it was his eyes were not open, for he was fast asleep, and dreaming that he was doing battle with the giant" [16].

polysomnographically confirmed RBD [17]. In a MSA cohort, 73% of the patients reported clinical features of RBD and in 88% of them the suspicion was polysomnographically confirmed [18].

A large proportion of patients with idiopathic RBD (iRBD) are susceptible to develop a synucleinopathy (18% in 5 years, 40% in 10 years, and 52% in 12 years) [9–11, 19]. In the last decade, many studies provided evidence that in some patients the onset of RBD may precede the appearance of daytime parkinsonian manifestations (e.g., motor signs and cognitive symptoms) by up to decades [20, 21], suggesting that RBD should no longer be considered a complication but a part of the prodromal phase of these disorders [22, 23]. Recent studies confirm this notion: in the Parkinson's Progression Markers Initiative study, possible RBD emerged in 25% of drug-naïve PD patients [24].

Most of the available studies reported that RBD is more common among males than females. This does not necessarily reflect an association of RBD with gender but possibly differences in the referral rates which are likely due to males having more frequently violent/prominent episodes of dream enactment than females.

Clinical Characteristics

In RBD, voluntary movements may be affected during sleep differently than during the day [25]. In the recent years, a number of studies focused not only on the nocturnal behavioral profile, but also on the daytime clinical characteristics of patients with RBD.

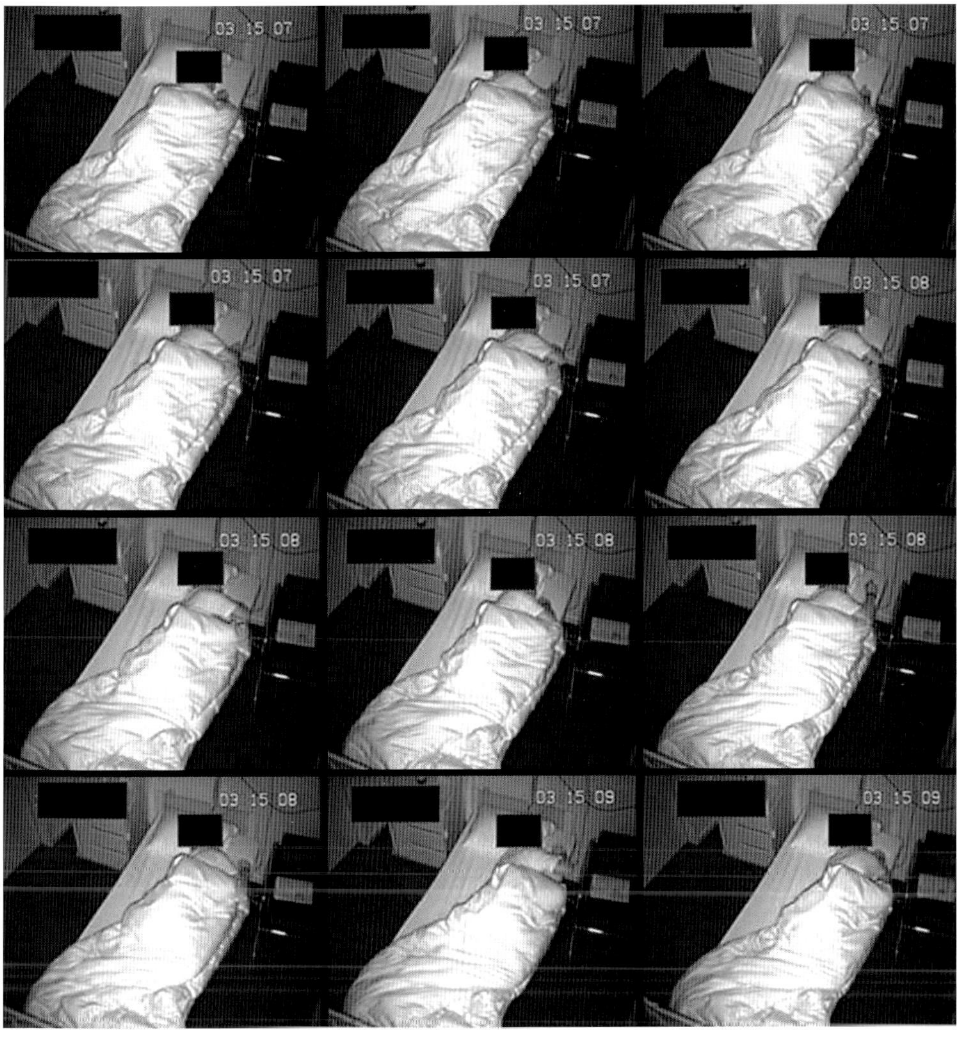

Fig. 2. Sequential frames recorded in a patient with multisystem atrophy and REM sleep behavior disorder, showing complex and semi-purposeful behavior during REM sleep.

Nocturnal Clinical Characteristics

Behaviors

Motor activities and behaviors in RBD range from slight hand movement and twitching of the extremities to kicking, grabbing, punching, talking, loud vocalization or screaming, and even complex, violent, and self-injurious behaviors (Fig. 2). Autonomic activation is limited/absent [9, 25].

Violent and self-injurious behaviors often pose a great social and emotional/mental distress to subjects with RBD and are frequently the reason for consultation or referral to a sleep center [26]. Self-protection measures taken by the patients to prevent injuries are not uncommon (Fig. 3).

In addition, the characteristic features of RBD provide a unique window into dreaming and the frequently accompanying violent behavior. The detailed research of the specific dream contents in RBD in combination with the increasing understanding of the loss of motor inhibition and the resulting "dream enactment" would offer great opportunities for scientist to deepen their knowledge about the organization/functions of dreaming and the cognitive and emotional processes occuring during dreaming.

Recently, genetically modified animals, characterized by a precise REM sleep-associated behavioral phenotype, were produced. From these animal models, we can gain more understanding (1) of the contribution of several factors, including genetics and epigenetics, to prevalence, clinical characteristics (e.g., nocturnal vs. daytime), and disease evolution and (2) of the role of brainstem and other supratentorial mechanisms to the underlying RBD pathophysiology. This should also help us to develop more sophisticated methods of early diagnosis and causative treatment of the disease.

References

1 Schenck CH, Bundlie SR, Patterson AL, et al: Rapid eye movement sleep behavior disorder. A treatable parasomnia affecting older adults. JAMA 1987;257: 1786–1789.

2 American Academy of Sleep Medicine.ICSD-2 – The Internatiomal Classification of Sleep Disorders, 2nd edtion. Westchester, IL, 2005.

3 Jouvet M, Vimont P, Delorme F: [Elective suppression of paradoxal sleep in the cat by monoamine oxidase inhibitors]. C R Seances Soc Biol Fil 1965;159: 1595–1599.

4 Chokroverty S, Allen RP, Walters AS: Sleep and Movement Disorders, 2 edition. Oxford University Press, 2013.

5 Passouant P, Cadilhac J, Ribstein M: [Sleep privation with eye movements using antidepressive agents]. Rev Neurol (Paris) 1972;127:173–192.

6 Tachibana M, Tanaka K, Hishikawa Y, Kaneko Z: A Sleep Study of Acute Psychotic States due to Alcohol and Meprobamate Addiction; in: Weitzman E, (ed): Advances in Sleep Research. New York, Spectrum, 1975, pp 177–203.

7 De Barros-Ferreira M, Chodkiewicz JP, Lairy GC, et al: Disorganized relations of tonic and phasic events of REM sleep in a case of brain-stem tumour. Electroencephalogr Clin Neurophysiol 1975;38:203–207.

8 Iranzo A, Santamaria J, de Riquer M: Sleep and sleep disorders in Don Quixote. Sleep Med 2004;5:97–100.

9 Videnovic A, Golombek D: Circadian and sleep disorders in Parkinson's disease. Exp Neurol 2013;243: 45–56.

10 Iranzo A, Molinuevo JL, Santamaria J, et al: Rapid-eye-movement sleep behaviour disorder as an early marker for a neurodegenerative disorder: a descriptive study. Lancet Neurol 2006;5:572–577.

11 Postuma RB, Gagnon JF, Vendette M, et al: Quantifying the risk of neurodegenerative disease in idiopathic REM sleep behavior disorder. Neurology 2009;72:1296–1300.

12 Mahlknecht P, Seppi K, Frauscher B, et al: Probable RBD and association with neurodegenerative disease markers: a population-based study. Mov Disord 2015;30:1417–1421.

13 Knudsen S, Gammeltoft S, Jennum PJ: Rapid eye movement sleep behaviour disorder in patients with narcolepsy is associated with hypocretin-1 deficiency. Brain 2010;133:568–579.

14 Di Fabio N, Poryazova R, Oberholzer M, et al: Sleepwalking, REM sleep behaviour disorder and overlap parasomnia in patients with Parkinson's disease. Eur Neurol 2013;70:297–303.

15 Mahowald MW, Schenck CH: Status dissociatus – a perspective on states of being. Sleep 1991;14:69–79.

16 De Cervantes: Don Quixote, Part I. Devoted Publishing, Woodstock, Ontario 2016, p 167.

17 Alatriste-Booth V, Rodriguez-Violante M, Camacho-Ordonez A, et al: Prevalence and correlates of sleep disorders in Parkinson's disease: a polysomnographic study. Arq Neuropsiquiatr 2015;73:241–245.

18 Palma JA, Fernandez-Cordon C, Coon EA, et al: Prevalence of REM sleep behavior disorder in multiple system atrophy: a multicenter study and meta-analysis. Clin Auton Res 2015;25:69–75.

19 Iranzo A, Tolosa E, Gelpi E, et al: Neurodegenerative disease status and post-mortem pathology in idiopathic rapid-eye-movement sleep behaviour disorder: an observational cohort study. Lancet Neurol 2013;12:443–453.
20 Iranzo A, Molinuevo JL, Santamaria J, et al: Rapid-eye-movement sleep behaviour disorder as an early marker for a neurodegenerative disorder: a descriptive study. Lancet Neurol 2006;5:572–577.
21 Claassen DO, Josephs KA, Ahlskog JE, et al: REM sleep behavior disorder preceding other aspects of synucleinopathies by up to half a century. Neurology 2010;75:494–499.
22 Postuma RB, Lang AE, Gagnon JF, et al: How does parkinsonism start? Prodromal parkinsonism motor changes in idiopathic REM sleep behaviour disorder. Brain 2012;135(pt 6):1860–1870.
23 Chaudhuri KR, Martinez-Martin P, Odin P, et al: Handbook of Non-Motor Symptoms in Parkinson's Disease. Springer Healthcare UK: Imprint: Springer Healthcare, Heidelberg, 2011, pp. XIII, 97.
24 Chahine LM, Xie SX, Simuni T, et al: Longitudinal changes in cognition in early Parkinson's disease patients with REM sleep behavior disorder. Parkinsonism Relat Disord 2016;27:102–106.
25 De Cock VC, Vidailhet M, Leu S, et al: Restoration of normal motor control in Parkinson's disease during REM sleep. Brain 2007;130(pt 2):450–456.
26 Olson EJ, Boeve BF, Silber MH: Rapid eye movement sleep behaviour disorder: demographic, clinical and laboratory findings in 93 cases. Brain 2000;123:331–339.
27 Fantini ML, Corona A, Clerici S, et al: Aggressive dream content without daytime aggressiveness in REM sleep behavior disorder. Neurology 2005;65:1010–1015.
28 Arnulf I, Neutel D, Herlin B, et al: Sleepiness in idiopathic REM sleep behavior disorder and Parkinson disease. Sleep 2015;38:1529–1535.
29 Montagna P, Chokroverty S: Sleep Disorders Part II, Series: Handbook of Clinical Neurology, Elsevier: 1 edition, 27 November, 2012, pp 874–875.
30 Ferini-Strambi L, Di Gioia MR, Castronovo V, et al: Neuropsychological assessment in idiopathic REM sleep behavior disorder (RBD): does the idiopathic form of RBD really exist? Neurology 2004;62:41–45.
31 Ferini-Strambi L, Marelli S, Galbiati A, et al: REM Sleep Behavior Disorder (RBD) as a marker of neurodegenerative disorders. Arch Ital Biol 2014;152:129–146.
32 Terzaghi M, Zucchella C, Rustioni V, et al: Cognitive performances and mild cognitive impairment in idiopathic rapid eye movement sleep behavior disorder: results of a longitudinal follow-up study. Sleep 2013;36:1527–1532.
33 Poryazova R, Oberholzer M, Baumann CR, et al: REM sleep behavior disorder in Parkinson's disease: a questionnaire-based survey. J Clin Sleep Med 2013;9:55–59.
34 Boeve BF: Pathophysiology of REM sleep behaviour disorder and relevance to neurodegenerative disease. Brain 2007;130:2770–2788.
35 Fraigne JJ, Torontali ZA, Snow MB, et al: REM sleep at its core – circuits, neurotransmitters, and pathophysiology. Front Neurol 2015;6:123.
36 Valencia Garcia S, Libourel PA, Lazarus M, et al: Genetic inactivation of glutamate neurons in the rat sublaterodorsal tegmental nucleus recapitulates REM sleep behaviour disorder. Brain 2017;140:414–428.
37 Eisensehr I, Linke R, Tatsch K, et al: Increased muscle activity during rapid eye movement sleep correlates with decrease of striatal presynaptic dopamine transporters. IPT and IBZM SPECT imaging in subclinical and clinically manifest idiopathic REM sleep behavior disorder, Parkinson's disease, and controls. Sleep 2003;26:507–512.
38 Dauvilliers Y, Postuma RB, Ferini-Strambi L, et al: Family history of idiopathic REM behavior disorder: a multicenter case-control study. Neurology 2013;80:2233–2235.
39 Gan-Or Z, Mirelman A, Postuma RB, et al: GBA mutations are associated with Rapid Eye Movement Sleep Behavior Disorder. Ann Clin Transl Neurol 2015;2:941–945.
40 Gan-Or Z, Montplaisir JY, Ross JP, et al: The dementia-associated APOE ε4 allele is not associated with rapid eye movement sleep behavior disorder. Neurobiol Aging 2017;49:218. e13–218. e15.
41 Sixel-Doring F, Zimmermann J, Wegener A, et al: The evolution of REM sleep behavior disorder in early Parkinson disease. Sleep 2016;39:1737–1742.
42 Mathis J, Hess CW, Bassetti C: Isolated mediotegmental lesion causing narcolepsy and rapid eye movement sleep behaviour disorder: a case evidencing a common pathway in narcolepsy and rapid eye movement sleep behaviour disorder. J Neurol Neurosurg Psychiatry 2007;78:427–429.
43 Iranzo A, et al: Rapid eye movement sleep behavior disorder and potassium channel antibody-associated limbic encephalitis. Ann Neurol 2006;59:178–181.
44 Schenck CH, Montplaisir JY, Frauscher B, et al: Rapid eye movement sleep behavior disorder: devising controlled active treatment studies for symptomatic and neuroprotective therapy – a consensus statement from the International Rapid Eye Movement Sleep Behavior Disorder Study Group. Sleep Med 2013;14:795–806.
45 Galbiati A, Rinaldi F, Giora E, et al: Behavioural and cognitive-behavioural treatments of parasomnias. Behav Neurol 2015;2015:786928.

46 Kunz D, Mahlberg R: A two-part, double-blind, placebo-controlled trial of exogenous melatonin in REM sleep behaviour disorder. J Sleep Res 2010;19: 591–596.
47 Schmidt MH, Koshal VB, Schmidt HS: Use of pramipexole in REM sleep behavior disorder: results from a case series. Sleep Med 2006;7:418–423.
48 Di Giacopo R, Fasano A, Quaranta D, et al: Rivastigmine as alternative treatment for refractory REM behavior disorder in Parkinson's disease. Mov Disord 2012;27:559–561.
49 Eugster L, Bargiotas P, Bassetti CL, et al: Deep brain stimulation and sleep-wake functions in Parkinson's disease: a systematic review. Parkinsonism Relat Disord 2016;32:12–19.

Prof. Claudio L.A. Bassetti, Chairman and Head
Neurology Department, Inselspital, Bern University Hospital
Freiburgstrasse 18
CH–3010 Bern (Switzerland)
E-Mail claudio.bassetti@insel.ch

Bogousslavsky J (ed): Neurologic-Psychiatric Syndromes in Focus. Part I – From Neurology to Psychiatry.
Front Neurol Neurosci. Basel, Karger, 2018, vol 41, pp 117–124 (DOI: 10.1159/000475702)

Charles Bonnet Syndrome and Other Hallucinatory Phenomena

François Boller[a] • Daniel S. Birnbaum[a] • Nicoletta Caputi[a, b]

[a]Department of Neurology, George Washington University Medical School, Washington, DC, USA;
[b]University of L'Aquila, Department of Life, Health and Environmental Science, L'Aquila, Italy

Abstract

Descriptions of hallucinatory phenomena have figured prominently since the beginning of recorded history. Jean Etienne Esquirol (1772–1840) is usually credited for having introduced the term in 1817, differentiating between hallucinations and illusions. Both are wrong perceptions, but in illusions, an external stimulus is always present whereas hallucinations are perceptions that occur in the absence of corresponding sensory stimuli. They occur in a variety of conditions but more often in the mentally ill, especially in schizophrenia where hallucinations, particularly auditory hallucinations represent for many, such as Henri Ey one of the cardinal features. This chapter, however, deals with visual hallucinations as found in individuals who are not necessarily mentally ill: the Charles Bonnet syndrome and autoscopy.

Introduction

The Charles Bonnet Syndrome

Jean Etienne Esquirol (1772–1840) is usually credited for having introduced the term hallucination in 1817 in the French Dictionary of the Medical Science [1] and for differentiating between hallucinations and illusions. Both are wrong perceptions, but hallucinations are perceptions that occur in "a mad person who has the thorough conviction of an actually perceived sensation, while no object suited to excite that sensation is present within the range of his senses," whereas in illusions, an external stimulus is always present.

Hallucinations may occur in a variety of medical conditions (psychiatric and neurodegenerative diseases, epilepsy, metabolic disorders, drug ingestion), but also in individuals without any illness. Charles Bonnet's descriptions of his grandfather in 1769 [2], Charles Lullin, highlighted that visual hallucinations could occur even in the absence of cognitive and psychiatric dysfunctions.

Lullin was an intelligent and articulate 89-year-old magistrate who started having subjective perception of silent visions of men, women, birds, carriages, and buildings, varying in size, shape, and place, occurring in association with visual deterioration after bilateral cataract surgery. His cognition was intact and he fully realized that his visions were "fictions" of his brain. As pointed out by Menon et al. [3] in their review, an irony of history saw Bonnet, deaf from the age of 7, himself suffering deterioration of vision early in life, followed by symptoms typical of the syndrome which now bears his name. However, it was not until 1936, when de Morsier recognized the scientific value of Bonnet's descriptions [4], that these phenomena were widely appreciated by the scientific community.

De Morsier was born in Paris where he spent part of his professional life training with Gaétan de Clérambault. However, he had Swiss origins and went to medical school in Geneva where he later became the first Chair of Neurology. Therefore, he knew about the work of his fellow country man, the Genevois Charles Bonnet and since then the eponym has stuck.

Another report describing the association of visual hallucinations with "lesions of the visual apparatus" was coincidentally published in the same year. While de Morsier was not well known and published in a "parochial Swiss journal", Jean Lhermitte was already a giant and he published in a major journal with De Ajuriaguerra who was later to also become a giant, together with Lhermitte's other "pupil," Henry Hécaen.

The Charles Bonnet syndrome (CBS) is usually defined as complex visual hallucinations occurring in individuals without cognitive or psychiatric diseases and with preserved intellectual functions and often associated with loss of visual acuity due to different ophthalmologic conditions (macular degeneration, glaucoma, cataracts). Recently, though, the CBS was described in a patient without vision loss or optic nerve atrophy who underwent a transsphenoidal adenomectomy for a pituitary macroadenoma and who experienced visual hallucination with his eyes closed [5].

Epidemiology

The prevalence is unknown, also because it is probably under-reported or under recognized. Menon et al. [3] indicate that elementary visual phenomena are found in 41–59% of patients with visual impairment. However, the complex hallucinations which constitute the CBS occur in 11–15% of people with visual impairment, either due to medical cause or artificially induced, for instance in preparation of cataract surgery. They are seen more often in people well into their 70s, but they have also been reported in children who experience rapid visual loss. There is no clear gender preponderance. Reported prevalence rates vary considerably: 6.4% in Turkey [6], between 0.47 and 15% in Spain [7], 1.4% in China [8], 8.3% in Denmark [9], 17.5% in Australia [10], 18.8% in Canada [11].

Diagnosis

De Morsier defined CBS as the occurrence of visual hallucinations in elderly people with intact cerebral function. He was, of course, aware of the frequent presence of ocular pathology, but he thought it was not the cause of the phenomenon and that it was not even obligatory, an aspect with which we agree. Later on, the definition was enlarged to mention that the hallucinations could be either persistent or recurring; that they are often pleasant, but occasionally may be frightening. And most importantly that the patients are often aware of the fact that there is no real stimulus present, thus leading to the name of pseudo-hallucinations. This preserved insight implies more or less intact cognitive functioning, as well as absence of altered consciousness, psychiatric disorders, sleep disorders or focal neurological lesions.

Although CBS has no official diagnostic criteria in general, features that can be used as guidelines include patients with loss of acuity (e.g., age-related macular degeneration, glaucoma, and cataract) who experienced at least one complex visual hallucination (none in other sensory modalities) and who preserve insight of the unreal nature of hallucinations.

Hallucinations vary in frequency, from once per year to several times a day, and in duration, from several hours to few seconds. In most cases, they occur on a daily basis and last a few minutes [12].

Content

Of course, content is quite varied. As written by Menon et al. [3]:

> "The most common image is that of a person. Other descriptions mention disembodied distorted faces, small costumed figures and branching structures; vivid images of animals and figures; subtle geometric forms; well defined complex figures and faces; Lilliputian (miniaturized), normal size and "larger-than life." Images; they can be black and white, but are more commonly in color, of varying degrees of complexity.
>
> These hallucinations are always localized in external space and the contents are well organized, defined, and brilliantly clear. In the context of coexistent visual impairment, the clarity of the visions contrasts sharply with the blurred perception of real objects.
>
> Patients may perceive visions of themselves, sometimes at an earlier stage of life, a phenomenon referred to as autoscopy (AP) (see below).
>
> Déjà vu experiences are uncommon. Subjects rarely recognize the figures as living or deceased acquaintances. Typically, the hallucinations are described as a sudden, sharply focused,

immobile image occurring with eyes open and often disappearing spontaneously within seconds. Alternatively they have been described as a solitary constant, solid object in the central visual field.

Atypical CBS hallucinations classified into atypical sensory-perceptual (ASP) or atypical psychodynamic (APD) varieties have also been described. APS hallucinations differ from typical complex visual hallucinations in one or more characteristics such as duration, movements, coordination, or participation of another sense (the latter widely considered an exclusion criterion for CBS). APD hallucinations, similar to dreams are more complex, mirroring the subject's psychological state, changing in content and frequency with alternations in the person's inner life or daily activities and may be repetitive."

Reports about movement vary considerably. Hallucinations are more often static but can also move either *en bloc* or partially, with parts of the image in motion within a static frame. The content is often stereotyped but can also vary from time to time. The duration varies from a few seconds to hours, sometimes disappearing only with sleep. On occasions, measures such as looking at them directly or engaging them in conversation can cause them to disappear. The coexistence with hallucinations in other modalities (mainly auditory) is no longer considered an exclusion criterion provided the subject retained insight into their unreality. Emotional distress, when present, is related more to the presence of hallucinations than to their content. The patient we described [13] would shout and swing at the snakes, yet she always stated that she knew they were "illusions." It is almost universally recognized that CBS is found in subjects with impaired vision. Very few [14] agree with the idea, like de Morsier, that visual dysfunction is not mandatory for diagnosis. On the contrary, hallucinations are often relieved by improvement of visual functions or, as was the case in our blind patient, by a neurosurgical procedure.

The Autoscopic Phenomena

Other visual hallucinatory conditions that may occur in healthy and diseased individuals are the autoscopic phenomena. As a phenomenon, AP has likely been with humanity even before the advent of scientific literature. This is evident by its frequent inclusion among religious experience, literature, movies, and even some culturally based medical experiences. Aristotle noted a gentleman named Antipheron who described his own mirror image appearing right before him, wherever he went [15]. The Bible makes reference to a possible out of body experience in 2 Corinthians 12:1–4. Specifically, AP is an often confused phenomenon that relates to (mis)perception and duplication of the self. The complexity of AP originates from its synthesis of multiple sensory inputs. Key sensory aspects include a sensation that the individual is (or is not) somewhere geographically different than the present physical location, visualizing the self-body (from within or externally), and identification that the observed object is actually the self. Variations can exist in that a single part of the body may be the focus of the autoscopic experience, although many would not consider this a truly autoscopic experience as it does not involve the whole body. Professor Olaf Blanke, currently of the École Polytechnique Fédérale of Lausanne, has been leading the investigation of AP for decades and in a 2005 paper helped define some of the current definitions related to AP. He mentions 3 terms, which will be addressed, including autoscopic hallucination (AH; seeing one's own body as if looking in a mirror), heautoscopy (the hallucination of feeling or seeing a presence or presences with one's own physical and psychological characteristics), and out of body experience (the hallucination of feeling one's own presence as outside one's own body, often floating nearby) [16].

These phenomena, as previously noted, have been extensively utilized in movies and literature. The Doppelgänger phenomena were particularly interesting for several authors, and the novelist Jean Paul Richter introduced the term in 1796. Unlike the comedy of errors, where the equivoques involve 2 twins, as in the *Menaechmi* by Plautus (III sec a.c.), the *Comedy of Errors* by Shakespeare (1590–1594), *I due gemelli veneziani* (The 2 Venetian twins) by Goldoni (1750), the autoscopic phenomena are conditions characterized by the hallucination of seeing one's own body.

Edgar Allan Poe in *William Wilson* (1839) wrote:

> "His name was the same as mine – William Wilson – although he did not belong to my family in any way. [...] My anger grew stronger with every happening that showed that William Wilson and I were alike, in body or in mind. I had not then discovered the surprising fact that we were of the same age; but I saw that we were of the same height, and I saw that in form and in face we were also much the same."

Another example can be found in The Double written by Dostoevsky (1846):

> "Sitting on his bed, also wearing a hat and coat, smiling slightly, puckering up his eyes and tipping him a friendly nod, was the stranger. Mr. Golyadkin wanted to scream, but could not – wanted to make some form of protest, but lacked the power. His hair stood on end, and he collapsed senseless with horror on the spot. And small wonder. He had fully recognized his friend of the night. It was none other than himself – Mr. Golyadkin ... Another Mr. Golyadkin, but exactly the same as him ... It was, in short, his double ... [.]"

The phenomenon was well represented also in famous movies, such as the *Duck Soup* (1933) starred by Marx Brothers or the *Twilight Zone* (1960) directed by John Brahm and written by Rod Serling, where Millicent Barnes sees her double in the train station.

In the same years in which the phenomenon was widely acknowledge by the fictional literature, Wigan [17] described the first medical case of a man who was seeing his double and who ended killing himself.

Disease Pathogenesis

The pathogenic localization of AP remains a topic of debate. However, a quick analysis of the phenomena will point the way towards some possibilities. There are significant visual, proprioceptive, vestibular, and identification components to AP. Both proprioception and vestibular senses are involved because the phenomena involve appreciation of where the body is in space (proprioception) as well as where the head is (vestibular input). As we know, the primary visual processing area is in the occipital cortex. Identification (faces, in particular) occurs at the junction of the inferior temporal lobe and the occipital lobe (fusiform gyrus). Sensory processing (including proprioception) occurs in the parietal lobe. The location of vestibular processing is less well known, but a 2012 meta-analysis of previous studies [18] suggests that the following areas are involved, including the retroinsular cortex, parietal operculum, and posterior insula. Other recent papers corroborate this approximate location as the region from which AP originate. A recent 2011 lesion analysis [19] suggests the nearby (continues as) temporo-parietal junction as the site that encodes self-location.

Other papers suggest that visual deficits are relevant, at least to autoscopic hallucination, and are mediated in part by the extrastriate cortex in the right occipital lobe. Heautoscopy may be mediated by the left posterior insula [20]. OBE was induced repetitively in a recent cortical stimulation study by stimulating the left TPJ [21]. As to what conditions can cause AP, the etiologies are as numerous as the potential sources of disorders of the brain and include epilepsy, migraine, neoplasia, infarction, infection, schizophrenia, depression, anxiety, and dissociative disorders [22].

Treatment and Management

No clear guidelines and universal treatment exist for the management of the CBS. Atypical antipsychotic medications such as Risperidone (Risperdal), Quetiapine (Seroquel), and Olanzapine (Zyprexa) have been used with varying success. Also, anticonvulsants (carbamazepine, clonazepam, valproate, gabapentin) have proved useful in some cases. Also, the underlying ophthalmic condition should be addressed and treated surgically if needed. Unfortunately, most of the studies are single case reports or they have inadequate description of sample and methodology. For these reasons there is insufficient justification for a standard treatment in CBS and it is recommended to use educational and practical interventions [23].

On the contrary, treatment of autoscopic phenomena, if needed, should relate to the underlying etiology.

Conclusions

In conclusion, physicians and ophthalmologist should be aware that visual hallucination may occur in patients without neurological and psychiatric conditions. Even if the CBS was recognized as a clinical entity 81 years ago and described even before, 2 main issues remain unresolved. First of all, there is a lack of well-defined clinical criteria that can be used for the diagnosis. Even the general agreement that marked loss in the acuity was necessary for the diagnosis, is now contested. This has led inevitably to a great heterogeneity that it is reflected in the variability of the detected prevalence and incidence. Secondly, the absence of large scale studies and the inadequate description of sample and methodology failed in confidently establishing an evidence-based treatment. In the future, double-blind, placebo-controlled clinical trials are needed to improve the management of this peculiar condition.

Further Reading

Ffytche DH: Visual hallucinatory syndromes: past, present, and future. Dialogues in Clinical Neuroscience 2006;9:173–189.

Anzellotti F, Onofrj V, Maruotti V, Ricciardi L, Franciotti R, Bonanni L, Thomas A, Onofrj M: Autoscopic phenomena: case report and review of literature. Behavioral and Brain Functions 2011; 7:1.

References

1 Esquirol E: Hallucinations. Dictionnaire des Sciences Médicales, par une Société de Médecins et de Chirurgiens, Panckoucke, Paris, 1817.

2 Bonnet C: Essai Analytique Sur Les Facultés De L'Ame: 6 (Vol. 6). Samuel Fauche, 1782.

3 Menon GJ, Rahman I, Menon SJ, Dutton GN: Complex visual hallucinations in the visually impaired: the Charles Bonnet Syndrome. Surv Ophthalmol 2003;48:58–72.

4 de Morsier G: Les sutomatismes visuels (Hallucinations visuelles retrochiasmatiques). Schweiz Med Wochenschr 1936;29:700–703.

5 Park JH, Ahn JH, Park JB, Joe S: Charles bonnet syndrome following trans-sphenoidal adenomectomy without optic nerve atrophy. Psychiatry Investig 2016;13:577–579.

6 Nalcaci S, İlim O, Oztas Z, Akkin C, Acarer A, Afrashi F, Mentes J: The prevalence and characteristics of charles bonnet syndrome in Turkish patients with retinal disease. Ophthalmologica 2016;236:48–52.

7 Santos-Bueso E, Sáenz-Francés F, Serrador-García M, Porta-Etessam J, Martínez-de-la-Casa JM, García-Feijoo J, García-Sánchez J: Prevalence and clinical characteristics of Charles Bonnet syndrome in Madrid, Spain. Eur J Ophthalmol 2014;24:960–963.

8 Hou Y, Zhang Y: The prevalence and clinical characteristics of Charles Bonnet syndrome in Chinese patients. Gen Hosp Psychiatry 2012;34:566–570.

9 Singh A, Sørensen TL: The prevalence and clinical characteristics of Charles Bonnet Syndrome in Danish patients with neovascular age-related macular degeneration. Acta Ophthalmol 2012;90:476–480.

10 Vukicevic M, Fitzmaurice K: Butterflies and black lacy patterns: the prevalence and characteristics of Charles Bonnet hallucinations in an Australian population. Clin Exp Ophthalmol 2008;36:659–665.

11 Gordon KD: Prevalence of visual hallucinations in a national low vision client population. Can J Ophthalmol 2016;51:3–6.

12 Teunisse RJ, Zitman FG, Cruysberg JR, Hoefnagels WH, Verbeek AL: Visual hallucinations in psychologically normal people: Charles Bonnet's syndrome. Lancet 1996;347:794–797.

13 McNamara ME, Heros RC, Boller F: Visual hallucinations in blindness: the Charles Bonnet syndrome. Int J Neurosci 1982;17:13–15.

14 Podoll K, Osterheider M, Noth J: Das Charles Bonnet-Syndrom. Fortschr Neurol Psychiatr 1989;57: 43–60.

15 Bicknell P: "Déjà vu, autoscopia, and antipheron: notes on aristotle, 'memory and recollection', i, 451a 8–12 and 'meteorologica', iii, 4, 373b 1–10." Acta Classica 1981;24:156–159.

16 Blanke O, Mohr C: Out-of-body experience, heautoscopy, and autoscopic hallucination of neurological origin implications for neurocognitive mechanisms of corporeal awareness and self-consciousness. Brain Res Brain Res Rev 2005;50:184–199.

17 Wigan AL: A New View of Insanity. The Duality of the Mind Proved by the Structure, Functions, and Diseases of the Brain, and by the Phenomena of Mental Derangement, and Shewn to be Essential to Moral Responsibility. Longman, 1844.

18 Lopez C, Blanke O, Mast FW: The human vestibular cortex revealed by coordinate-based activation likelihood estimation meta-analysis. Neuroscience 2012; 212:159–179.
19 Ionta S, Heydrich L, Lenggenhager B, Mouthon M, Fornari E, Chapuis D, Gassert R, Blanke O: Multisensory mechanisms in temporo-parietal cortex support self-location and first-person perspective. Neuron 2011;70:363–374.
20 Heydrich L, Blanke O: Distinct illusory own-body perceptions caused by damage to posterior insula and extrastriate cortex. Brain 2013;136(pt 3):790–803.
21 Bos EM, Spoor JK, Smits M, Schouten JW, Vincent AJ: Out-of-body experience during awake craniotomy. World Neurosurg 2016;92:e9–e86.e13.
22 Blanke O, Landis T, Spinelli L, Seeck M: Out-of-body experience and autoscopy of neurological origin. Brain 2004;127(pt 2):243–258.
23 Hughes DF: Charles Bonnet syndrome: a literature review into diagnostic criteria, treatment and implications for nursing practice. J Psychiatr Ment Health Nurs 2013;20:169–175.

François Boller, MD, PhD, Professor of Neurology
Department of Neurology, George Washington University Medical School
2150 Pennsylvania Avenue NW, Suite 9–400
Washington, DC 20037 (USA)
E-Mail fboller@mfa.gwu.edu

Author Index

Subject Index